From Immigration Controls to Welfare Controls

This edited collection addresses theoretical, political and practical aspects of the connection between external immigration controls and internal welfare controls. It considers the implications for both those subject to controls and those drawn into the web of implementing internal welfare controls. Topics discussed include:

- forced dispersal of asylum seekers
- local authority and voluntary sector regulations
- nationalism, racism, class and 'fairness'
- strategies for resistance to controls
- controls in the USA

The book engages with the debates thrown up by the struggles of migrants, refugees and anti-racists, straddling the barrier which often exists between academic and political debates. It provides support to those unwittingly drawn into administering controls, showing how the role of welfare workers as immigration control enforcers is not a sudden imposition, but has existed since the introduction of controls in 1905.

From Immigration Controls to Welfare Controls will provide a valuable resource for all those professionals who come into contact with the issues surrounding immigration.

Steve Cohen is former Co-ordinator of Greater Manchester Immigration Unit, **Beth Humphries** is Reader in Social Work, Lancaster University and **Ed Mynott** is Research Fellow, Centre for European Political Communications, Leeds University.

D0097105

The State of Welfare
Edited by Mary Langan

Throughout the Western world, welfare states are in transition. Changing social, economic and political circumstances have rendered obsolete the systems that emerged in the 1940s out of the experiences of depression, war and social conflict. New structures of welfare are now taking shape in response to the conditions of today: globalisation and individuation, the demise of traditional allegiances and institutions, the rise of new forms of identity and solidarity.

In Britain, the New Labour government has linked the projects of implementing a new welfare settlement and forging a new moral purpose in society. Enforcing 'welfare to work', on the one hand, and tackling 'social exclusion' on the other, the government aims to rebalance the rights and duties of citizens and redefine the concept of equality.

The State of Welfare series provides a forum for the debate about the new shape of welfare into the millennium.

Titles of related interest also in *The State of Welfare* series:

From Immigration Controls to Welfare Controls

**Edited by
Steve Cohen, Beth Humphries
and Ed Mynott**

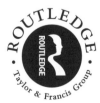

London and New York

First published 2002
by Routledge
11 New Fetter Lane, London EC4P 4EE

Simultaneously published in the USA and Canada
by Routledge
29 West 35th Street, New York, NY 10001

Routledge is an imprint of the Taylor & Francis Group

Selection and editorial matter © 2002 Steve Cohen, Beth
Humphries and Ed Mynott

Individual chapters © 2002 individual contributors

Typeset in Times by
M Rules
Printed and bound in Great Britain by
Biddles Ltd, Guildford and King's Lynn

All rights reserved. No part of this book may be reprinted or
reproduced or utilised in any form or by any electronic,
mechanical, or other means, now known or hereafter
invented, including photocopying and recording, or in any
information storage or retrieval system, without permission in
writing from the publishers.

British Library Cataloguing in Publication Data
A catalogue record for this book is available from the British
Library

Library of Congress Cataloging in Publication Data
A catalog record for this book has been requested

ISBN 0–415–25082–X (hbk)
ISBN 0–415–25083–8 (pbk)

Contents

Series editor's preface

State welfare policies reflect changing perceptions of key sources of social instability. In the first half of the twentieth century – from Bismarck to Beveridge – the welfare state emerged as a set of policies and institutions which were – in the main – a response to the 'problem of labour', the threat of class conflict. The major objective was to contain and integrate the labour movement. In the post-war decades, as this threat receded, the welfare state became consolidated as a major employer and provider of a wide range of services and benefits to every section of society. Indeed, it increasingly became the focus of blame for economic decline and was condemned for its inefficiency and ineffectiveness.

Since the end of the Cold War, the major fear of capitalist societies is no longer class conflict, but the socially disintegrative consequences of the system itself. Increasing fears and anxieties about social instability – including unemployment and homelessness, delinquency, drug abuse and crime, divorce, single parenthood and child abuse – reflect deep-seated apprehensions about the future of modern society.

The role of state social policy in the Clinton–Blair era is to restrain and regulate the destructive effects of market forces, symbolised by the Reagan–Thatcher years. On both sides of the Atlantic, governments have rejected the old polarities of left and right, the goals of both comprehensive state intervention and rampant free-market individualism. In its pursuit of a 'third way' the New Labour government, which came to power in Britain in May 1997, has sought to define a new role for government at a time when politics has largely retreated from its traditional concerns about the nature and direction of society.

What are the values of the third way? According to Tony Blair, the people of middle England 'distrust heavy ideology', but want 'security and stability'; they 'want to refashion the bonds of community life' and, 'although they believe in the market economy, they do not believe that the only values that matter are those of the market place' (*The Times*, 25 July 1998). The values of the third way reflect and shape a traditional and conservative response to the dynamic and unpredictable world of the late 1990s.

The view expressed by Michael Jacobs, a leading participant in the revived Fabian Society, that 'we live in a strongly individualised society which is falling apart' is widely shared (*The Third Way*, London: The Fabian Society, 1998). For him, 'the fundamental principle' of the third way is 'to balance the autonomous demands of the individual with the need for social cohesion or "community".' A key New Labour concept that follows from this preoccupation with community is that of 'social exclusion'. Proclaimed the government's 'most important innovation' when it was announced in August 1997, the 'social exclusion unit' is at the heart of New Labour's flagship social policy initiative – the 'welfare to work' programme. The preoccupation with 'social exclusion' indicates a concern about tendencies towards fragmentation in society and a self-conscious commitment to policies which seek to integrate atomised individuals and thus to enhance social cohesion.

The popularity of the concept of social exclusion reflects a striking tendency to aggregate diverse issues so as to imply a common origin. The concept of social exclusion legitimises the moralising dynamic of New Labour. Initiatives such as 'welfare to work', targeting the young unemployed and single mothers, emphasise individual responsibility. Duties – to work, to save, to adopt a healthy lifestyle, to do homework, to 'parent' in the approved manner – are the common themes of New Labour social policy; obligations take precedence over rights.

Though the concept of social exclusion targets a smaller section of society than earlier categories such as 'the poor' or 'the underclass', it does so in a way which does imply a societal responsibility for the problems of fragmentation, as well as indicating a concern to draw people back – from truancy, sleeping rough, delinquency and drugs, etc. – into the mainstream of society. Yet New Labour's sympathy for the excluded only extends as far as the provision of voluntary work and training schemes, parenting classes and drug rehabilitation programmes. The socially excluded are no longer allowed to be the passive recipients of benefits; they are obliged to participate in their moral reintegration. Those who refuse to subject themselves to these apparently benign forms of regulation may soon find themselves the target of more coercive interventions.

There is a further dimension to the third way. The very novelty of New Labour initiatives necessitates the appointment of new personnel and the creation of new institutions to overcome the inertia of the established structures of central and local government. To emphasize the importance of its drugs policy, the government has created the new office of Drugs Commissioner – 'Tsar' – and prefers to implement the policy through a plethora of voluntary organisations, rather than through traditional channels. Health action zones, education action zones and employment action zones are the chosen vehicles for policy innovation in their respective areas. At higher levels of government, semi-detached special policy units, think tanks and quangos play an increasingly important role.

The State of Welfare series aims to provide a critical assessment of social policy in the new millennium. We will consider the new and emerging 'third way' welfare policies and practices and the way these are shaped by wider social and economic changes. Globalisation, the emergence of post-industrial society, the transformation of work, demographic shifts and changes in gender roles and family structures all have major consequences for patterns of welfare provision.

Social policy will also be affected by the demands of social movements – women, minority ethnic groups, disabled people – as well as groups concerned with sexuality or the environment. *The State of Welfare* series will examine these influences when analysing welfare practices in the first decade of the new millennium.

Mary Langan
February 1999

Contributors

Steve Cohen is an immigration lawyer, former co-ordinator of Greater Manchester Immigration Aid Unit and the author of *Immigration Controls, the Family and the Welfare State*. He is politically opposed to the existence of controls and to all notions that there can be 'fair' or 'just' or 'non-racist' controls. He has been involved in anti-deportation campaigns and in defence of asylum seekers for over 25 years, and considers it important that studies about immigration controls should be of value to these campaigns. He is about to embark on a study of the role, or otherwise, of the trade union movement in fighting for the right of entry into the UK of Jewish refugees fleeing Nazi Germany.

Michael Fix is a lawyer and principal research associate at the Urban Institute in Washington, DC, where he directs the Immigration Studies Program. The focus of his work in recent years has been in areas of immigration and civil rights policy. He has written or edited numerous books including, *Overlooked and Underserved: immigrant secondary students in US schools* (2000) and *Poverty Amid Prosperity: immigration and the changing face of rural California* (1997). He is currently directing a large study of the effects of welfare reform on immigrants in Los Angeles and New York.

Alison Harvey qualified as a barrister and holds a Masters degree in Human Rights Law. She is the Advocacy Officer at the medical Foundation for the Care of Victims of Torture in London, where she works to put forward the views of the Foundation on asylum at domestic, European and international levels. Alison has worked representing individual asylum seekers and as a researcher in the field of asylum. She is a trustee of Asylum Aid, a charity providing free representation to asylum seekers, and an editor of *Butterworths Immigration Law Service*. She is an expert on the legislative framework of the new support arrangements and on their implementation.

Debra Hayes is a senior lecturer in social work in the Department of Applied Community Studies at Manchester Metropolitan University. She worked in the Probation Service for seven years prior to this. During that time she began collaborating with the Greater Manchester Immigration Aid Unit concerning the deportation of black prisoners, or 'double punishment'. She has been involved on behalf of the university, in organising three national conferences on prisoners and deportation, children, social work and immigration, and on health and immigration control. Since then her research, publications and curriculum development have concerned the relationship between welfare and immigration control. She is an active socialist and remains involved in local campaigns to defend asylum seekers and stop deportation.

Beth Humphries has been an academic and researcher for many years, after having been a social worker in the UK, in the statutory and voluntary sectors. She has published in the fields of research methods and social work, and has for the past seven years carried out research in the area of immigration controls and welfare. She is a former member of the management committee of the Greater Manchester Immigration Aid Unit. Her publications include a study on changes in the NHS related to the immigration status of patients (with Steve Cohen and others), and one on the needs of separated young asylum seekers (with Ed Mynott). She is currently Reader in Social Work at Lancaster University.

Adele Jones is a lecturer in social work at the University of the West Indies, Republic of Trinidad and Tabago. She has worked on research projects examining issues related to young black carers, young black people and homelessness, and an international study of innovative family support. Previous research and development work has focused on residential care, child protection and work with young black disabled people. Her most recent research was an examination of immigration issues for children and young people. She has also published on child protection and theory in social work research.

Shirley Joshi teaches sociology at the University of Central England where she is course director for the MA/Diploma in Immigration Policy, Law and Practice. She has been involved in campaigns against racist immigration laws and in organisations delivering a service to immigrants, asylum seekers and refugees for the last 40 years.

Ed Mynott works as a researcher in the Department of Applied Community Studies at Manchester Metropolitan University. His current fields of research and publication are immigration, asylum and welfare. He gained his PhD at the University of Manchester in 1995 with a study of the 'social purity' movement in Victorian Britain. He has been involved in a range of political campaigns since the 1980s, particularly against deportations and in defence of asylum seekers. He is a long standing member of the Socialist Workers Party.

Terry Patterson is a member of the Committee for Non-Racist Benefits. He is a welfare rights and housing practitioner, trainer researcher and author. His writings on social entitlements and equality issues range from *Survival Guide to London for Young Homeless People* (Centrepoint 1981) to 'Welfare rights advice and the new materialism', 2001, in *Benefits*, 30: 5–10, and with Dean Herd, 'Poor Manchester: old problems and New Deals', in J. Peck and K Ward (eds) (2001) *City of Revolution: restructuring Manchester.* Manchester: Manchester University Press.

Wendy Zimmermann is a senior research associate at the Urban Institute in Washington, DC, specialising in immigration policy and immigrant integration. She has focused most of her recent work on the impact of welfare reform on immigrants and their families, including looking at how states in the USA have responded to their new authority to limit immigrants' access to the safety net. Her recent publications include *Patchwork Policies: state assistance for immigrants under welfare reform* (with Karen Tumlin), and *The Integration of Immigrant Families in the United States* (with Michael Fix).

Acknowledgements

Our thanks are due to the contributors to the volume, who recognised the importance of increasing the range of literature informing welfare practitioners and others of how immigration controls impinge increasingly on their work. All of them took time in busy jobs to produce their chapters, and responded with good humour and efficiency to the extra demands we made of them. Thanks too to Claire Faichnie for her help in the final stages of editing, and to Tony Openshaw of the National Coalition of Anti-Deportation Campaigns, who helped with permission related to the book's cover photograph. Our thanks are also due to Routledge and *State of Welfare* series editor, Mary Langan, for agreeing to publish the book, and to our contact at Routledge, Michelle Bacca.

Steve Cohen would like to thank his mum and dad to whose memory his political contribution is dedicated. He would also like to thank Tomas, Rachel, Fintan and Ellen, for being there.

Beth Humphries would particularly like to thank her co-editors Steve Cohen and Ed Mynott, and to express her admiration for their erudition, perseverance and political commitment in the face of many other important things happening in their lives! She is also, as ever, grateful for Marion's continuing support and interest in all her work.

Ed Mynott would also like to thank his co-editors for their hard work and forbearance. He would also like to thank all his comrades and colleagues, too numerous to name, whose collective intellectual and political contributions over the years have been vital in shaping his own thought.

1 Introduction

Locating the debate

Ed Mynott, Beth Humphries and Steve Cohen

This book has been written in the shadow of the Immigration and Asylum Act (1999), implemented by Britain's Labour government. This shocking legislation built on the worst elements of UK immigration policy, introducing a voucher system in place of cash benefits, a national system of forced dispersal, and was accompanied by an increased use of detention centres.

Britain is not alone in the direction of its policy. The construction of Fortress Europe and the increase in immigration controls in the United States (and elsewhere) has subjected human beings to appalling and degrading treatment, criminalising them for crossing borders. Thousands of migrants every year are paying the ultimate price for trying to move. Such was the plight of the 3000 people who are estimated to have died in the Gibraltar strait in the five years up to 2000 (Carroll 2000; Harding 2000). Mike Davis has described the result of President Clinton's unilateral militarisation of the border between Mexico and the United States in 1994: 'In the NAFTA [North Atlantic Free Trade Area] era, capital, like pollution, may flow freely across the border, but labor migration faces unprecedented criminalization and repression' (Davis 2000: 34). One recent study has estimated that nearly 1600 people had died as a result of the militarisation of the border (cited in Davis 2000: 34). This brutal reality was brought home to those of us living in Britain on 18 June 2000 as news broke that 58 Chinese people had suffocated to death in the back of a container truck in their desperate attempt to enter the UK.

However, there is more to the process of tightening controls than closing borders. Across the developed capitalist countries immigration control has increasingly come to involve the restriction of access to welfare provision on the grounds of immigration status. This collection of writings was brought together because we believed that a book was necessary which dealt with the connection between immigration control and welfare control. Any examination of this area quickly reveals that the connection has long been present. The current harmonisation across the European Union of policies to restrict asylum seekers' access to welfare – of which Britain's Immigration and Asylum Act is part – represents an intensification of the connection between immigration control and welfare control, not its creation.

Examining this area also throws light on a problematic characteristic of the welfare state. In particular it reveals how nationalism has justified the exclusion of certain people from access to provision. This exclusion cuts across the universalism and extension of social support more usually associated with the development of the welfare state.

This book takes sides. It aims to engage with the debates thrown up by the struggles of migrants, refugees and anti-racists. It takes a partisan position of support for those who are on the receiving end of the refined tortures of the asylum support system and those working within welfare provision who wish to resist the discrimination and racism which it entails and perpetuates.

The book also aims to straddle the barrier which often exists between academic and political debates, preferring to be an intervention into both. That requires being theoretically rigorous while also having something to say about the immediate contradictions, cruelties and dilemmas of immigration policy. The editors of this book (although not agreeing on everything) have sought to ground their criticism of current asylum regimes in an opposition to immigration controls. Indeed, while all contributors have their own perspective, it is opposition to all immigration controls, and a rejection of the utopian position that it is possible to construct fair or non-racist immigration controls, which has brought the editors together.

Our influences

There is a considerable literature on issues of immigration and racism which include discussion about British immigration controls. Some of the milestones in this literature are Foot (1965); Castles and Kosack (1973); Sivanandan (1982); Miles and Phizacklea (1984); Layton-Henry (1992) and Hayter (2000). It was during the 1980s that the link between immigration control and welfare was taken up by grass roots immigration advice and welfare advice bodies. Various publications appeared such as the *No Pass Laws Here Bulletin* and the influential Child Poverty Action Group pamphlet *Passport To Benefits?* (Gordon and Newnham 1985). The same year saw the publication of Paul Gordon's *Policing Immigration Controls* which was the last book (as opposed to pamphlet or article) for some time to deal in any depth with internal immigration controls and the link with welfare. Gordon argued that internal controls should be defined as 'any aspect of law or administration related in any way to immigration status which operates *within* the UK' (Gordon 1985: 2). His discussion included the more obvious aspects of control, the measures to trace and apprehend those who may be in breach of immigration laws. But it also covered the 'relationship between immigration law and other areas such as employment, housing and the welfare state'. Gordon made clear the result of making access to work and welfare dependent on immigration status: 'the overall effect is the questioning, restricting and controlling of rights, not just of those who are immigrants, but those who are commonly assumed to be, because they are black' (Gordon 1985: 2).

Work such as Gordon's popularised the understanding that internal immigration controls are likely to cast suspicion on all black people regardless of their immigration status. Organisations like the Committee for Non-Racist Benefits took up the question of racial discrimination in social security, and extensive research highlighted the reality of such discrimination. However, whilst this important effect was identified (the effect of racism), less attention has been paid to the continually developing system of internal controls which create and re-create this linkage, in the asylum and immigration legislation of the 1990s. It is only very recently that the connection between immigration control and welfare has begun to be analysed again in any depth, albeit from rather different perspectives (Bommes and Geddes 2000; Geddes 2000; Cohen 2001).

The removal of certain categories of asylum seeker from access to the welfare system was central to the asylum legislation of the 1990s. While this has been the subject of journalistic and political comment, and dealt with in reports mainly by the voluntary sector, it has not been the subject of sustained academic work – with the exception of the journal *Race and Class* (see especially Fekete 1998). Labour's Immigration and Asylum Act represents a leap forward in the removal of access to welfare. What has often gone unnoticed is that it is not simply asylum seekers but *every* person 'subject to immigration control' who has been removed from legal entitlement to a vast swathe of welfare provision. It is the huge amounts of benefits and services now dependent on immigration status for eligibility (and the new poor law created for asylum seekers) that represents such a significant and recent extension of internal controls as they relate to welfare provision.

There *is* already a literature which deals with the reception and settlement of refugees. In Britain, the Home Office has produced several research papers (Jones 1982; Carey-Wood *et al*. 1995; Duke and Marshall 1995; Field 1985). There are various books and articles about the experience of Vietnamese refugees in Britain (Joly 1988; Bell and Clinton 1992). Joly (1996) has written about reception and settlement policies, comparing the experiences of Chilean and Vietnamese refugees in the 1970s and 1980s in Britain and France, and specifically on local authority policy on refugees in Britain. Joly and Cohen (1989) bring together contributions covering many European countries and have as one of their major themes, 'the role of the state in the admission of refugees and its role, together with local authorities, in their settlement' (Joly and Cohen 1989: 9). Similar themes are amongst those addressed by Kushner and Knox (1999) in their definitive account of the refugee experience in the twentieth century.

This literature certainly reveals how problematic have been attempts by the state to include and 'integrate' those on whom it has bestowed the right to remain in Britain. However, the perspective of our book is not that of refugee reception and settlement as such – although that cannot fail to be deeply affected by a restrictive asylum policy, whatever the attempts by government to segregate the two issues (Home Office 2000).

The perspective of this book is the treatment of those who are subject to immigration control and the creation of regimes which deliberately categorise them as less deserving of social support than other people. Our intention has been to develop the theme of how governments have extended internal controls, particularly with reference to welfare provision. We have also highlighted the ways in which those who work within the welfare system are increasingly being drawn into systems of immigration control. We aim to encourage welfare workers and professionals to question these developments, and ask whether there is any prospect of resistance to these developments and what strategies might be used.

The structure of the book

The book is divided into three parts. Part I deals with political, historical and international issues. Part II deals with the contemporary issues in immigration and welfare. Part III goes from theory to resistance.

In Chapter 2 (which begins Part I) Ed Mynott uses a Marxist framework to look at how a racialised nationalism has been a constant driving force in the construction of immigration controls under capitalism. He also contrasts the immigration control/welfare link in the period of the welfare state's construction with today's period of its neoliberal restructuring. He concludes with a call for the 'creative fusion' of the established anti-racist and the new anti-capitalist movements.

In Chapter 3, Debra Hayes examines the history of the relationship between immigration controls and access to welfare in a British context. She traces its origins to the 1905 Aliens Act and the debates which preceded it. She explores how the theme of controlling access to welfare by immigration status developed throughout the twentieth century, with modern day asylum seekers becoming the equivalent of their 'alien' forebears.

In Chapter 4, Shirley Joshi tackles the class nature of British immigration controls from the Commonwealth Immigrants Act of 1962 to the present day. She notes the similarities between the racist underclass theories – prevalent in the United States – which stress welfare dependency – and the similar allegations which have regularly informed British immigration legislation. She concludes that Britain's current immigration policy is still underpinned by a discourse on the underclass as well as a moral panic about migrants.

In Chapter 5, Wendy Zimmermann and Michael Fix look at immigration and welfare reforms in the United States through the lens of mixed-status families. This provides a welcome opportunity to look at a relatively unexplored area, but one which could become important in British as well as United States immigration law. For example, there already exists in UK law the situation where one parent may be able to claim child benefit, but the other parent may not have the appropriate immigration status. Quite complex welfare or immigration problems in this respect can also arise in respect to Working Families Tax Credit and Council Tax or Housing Benefit. The question of mixed-immigration-status families is, as outlined in this chapter, significant in the USA because of children having US citizenship while their parents do not. By contrast, since 1983 birth in the UK has not led automatically to British citizenship. However, difference in immigration status between parents may be the next stage in the curtailing of benefit eligibility, with the state insisting both have the same appropriate status.

Part II, contemporary issues in immigration and welfare, begins with Chapter 6, in which Adele Jones examines how the pursuit of immigration controls impacts on family life. While acknowledging that the concept of the family is problematic, she shows that the limited commitment of the British government to supporting families is not extended to families subject to immigration controls. The principal legislative and policy provisions for the support of family life are then summarised. She concludes that there has been little attempt in social work literature, policy or practice to challenge or deconstruct the contradictions tacit in the privileging of immigration law over child care law.

In Chapter 7, Ed Mynott traces the evolution of social support systems for asylum seekers, from the shambles created by Britain's 1996 Asylum and Immigration Act to the new apartheid in welfare provision established by the 1999 Immigration and Asylum Act. He examines the impact of vouchers and the forced dispersal system. He questions the justifications given for local authorities' co-operation with dispersal and suggests some key issues for those resisting the dispersal and voucher systems.

In Chapter 8, Beth Humphries traces a slide from welfare to authoritarianism. She uses social work as an example of where the Home Office has attempted to enlist welfare professionals in the implementation of immigration controls. She analyses the contradictory role of social work with its ambivalence between 'care' and a disciplinary function, before suggesting that welfare professionals should be concerned less with efficiency than with ethics, politics and strategies of resistance.

In Chapter 9, Steve Cohen identifies a novel aspect of the 1999 Act and its implementation: the engagement of parts of the voluntary sector in a system which is directly antagonistic to the interests of refugees. In becoming a junior partner of the Home Office, they are dining with the devil. He argues that part of the voluntary sector is becoming a designated poor law enforcer and calls for non-cooperation by the voluntary sector with the new poor law, linked to a campaign for the reinstatement of welfare provision for asylum seekers.

In Chapter 10, Terry Patterson charts the insidious growth of forms of immigration control, residence and asylum seeker restrictions in social security provision over the last two decades in Britain, from the perspective of welfare rights advice. He looks at how policies were justified and received; their consequences for claimants, communities, advisers and staff; and the effectiveness of challenges to the changes. He concludes that human rights arguments mark the likely way ahead in face of the fortress mentalities of politicians in Britain and Europe who have institutionalised exclusion from welfare entitlement, racism and the culture of suspicion.

Part III, from theory to resistance, opens with Chapter 11, a legal view from Alison Harvey on how to challenge the 1999 Immigration and Asylum Act. She dissects the exclusion provisions of its Part VI which is at the heart of the legislation. She examines the potential to challenge exclusion from the welfare state; to challenge the operation of the national asylum support scheme; and to extend the ambit of that scheme. She recognises the Human Rights Act as a powerful tool – though not the only one. She suggests that legal challenges would test our commitment to human rights and welfare legislation, which, if successful, could be used to benefit all within Britain, not only those under immigration control.

In Chapter 12, Beth Humphries examines both the case for 'fair' immigration controls and the arguments entailed in anti-immigration control positions. She argues that an unfair system cannot be made fair, but that many of the contrary arguments make unintended concessions to those who advocate controls. Opponents of immigration controls need to use arguments which are not at risk of appropriation by those who support controls. She concludes that an absence of controls would not provide a panacea for all ills, but it would be a major structural shift, signalling a genuine commitment to an anti-racist world.

Finally, in Chapter 13, Steve Cohen puts forward some strategies for resistance. Because of the growing synthesis between welfare entitlements and immigration status, struggles are now taking place not only over the right to enter or remain, but over issues of welfare. Thus there is a more vital need than ever for a political alliance between those threatened by immigration controls and workers within welfare – an alliance which involves those workers' unions is more vital than ever. Such an alliance could resist the convergence of immigration controls with welfare controls.

The book is intended for academics, activists and people facing the injustice of immigration controls. We hope it will fulfil this aim and add to a growing literature in this field.

References

Bell, J. and Clinton, L. (1992) *The Unheard Community: a look at the housing conditions and needs of refugees from Vietnam living in London*, London: Refugee Action.

Bommes, M. and Geddes, A. (eds) (2000) *Welfare and Immigration: challenging the borders of the welfare state*, London: Routledge.

Carey-Wood, J., Duke, K., Karn, V. and Marshall, T. (1995) *The Settlement of Refugees in Britain. Home Office Research Study 141*, London: Home Office.

Carroll, R. (2000) 'In Praise of Smugglers' *The Guardian*, 2 September.

Castles, S. and Kosack, G. (1973) *Immigrant Workers and Class Structure in Western Europe*, London: Oxford University Press for the Institute of Race Relations.

Cohen, S. (2001) *Immigration Controls, the Family and the Welfare State: a handbook of law, theory, politics, and practice for local authority, voluntary sector and welfare state workers and legal advisors*, London: Jessica Kingsley.

——(1987) *It's the Same Old Story*, Manchester: Manchester City Council.

Davis, M. (2000) *Magical Urbanism: Latinos reinvent the US city*, London: Verso.

8   *Ed Mynott, Beth Humphries and Steve Cohen*

Duke, K. and Marshall, T. (1995) *Vietnamese Refugees since 1982. Home Office Research Study 142*, London: Home Office.

Fekete L. (1998) 'Blackening the economy: the path to convergence' *Race and Class*, 39(4): 1–22.

Field, S. (1985) *Resettling Refugees: the lessons of research. Home Office Research Study 87*, London: Home Office.

Foot, P. (1965) *Immigration and Race in British Politics*, Harmondsworth: Penguin.

Gordon, P. (1985) *Policing Immigration Controls: Britain's internal controls*, London: Pluto Press.

Gordon, P. and Newnham, A. (1985) *Passport to Benefits? Racism in Social Security*, London: Child Poverty Action Group and The Runnymede Trust.

Harding, J. (2000) *The Uninvited: refugees at the rich man's gate*, London: Profile Books.

Hayter, T. (2000) *Open Borders: the case against immigration controls*, London: Pluto Press.

Home Office (2000) *Full and Equal Citizens: a strategy for the integration of refugees into the United Kingdom*, London: Home Office.

Joly, D. and Cohen, R. (eds) (1989) *Reluctant Hosts: Europe and its refugees*, Aldershot: Avebury.

Jones, P. (1982) *Vietnamese Refugees. Home Office Research and Planning Unit Paper 13*, London: Home Office.

Kushner, T. and Knox, K. (1999) *Refugees in an Age of Genocide: global, national and local perspectives during the twentieth century*, London: Frank Cass.

Layton-Henry, Z. (1992) *The Politics of Immigration*, Oxford: Blackwell Publishers, 1992.

Miles, R. and Phizacklea, A. (1984) *White Man's Country: racism in British politics,* London: Pluto Press.

Sivanandan, A (1982) *A Different Hunger: writings on black resistance,* London: Pluto Press.

Part I

Political, historical and international issues

2 Nationalism, racism and immigration control

From anti-racism to anti-capitalism

Ed Mynott

It is almost a century since the first systematic immigration controls appeared in Britain and almost 40 years since the first controls on black people from Commonwealth countries. What has remained constant since then – and since the 1970s across Europe – is a stress by governments on the pressing need to control immigration.

Yet in reality, only certain immigrants have been targeted by immigration controls. At the beginning of the twentieth century it tended to be Jewish people fleeing Russia and eastern Europe. After the Second World War, it was black Commonwealth citizens in Britain, and black and third world migrants more generally across Europe and the United States. Since the mid-1980s, 'bogus' or 'abusive' asylum seekers (which, in the eyes of governments, turns out to be most of them) have moved to the forefront of the demonisation of third world migrants across the European Union.

At the same time, it is important to understand that the reality of migration is much broader and more complex than the rhetoric of immigration control would allow for. This was always true historically and remains true today (Castles and Miller 1998; Stalker 2000). There are many types of migration which are rarely viewed as problematic. For example, the Treaty of Rome guarantees nationals of what is now the European Union (although not all those within its borders) the freedom to seek and take up work and residence in any other member state (Ford 1994). Many have done so – in the main, white Europeans. Perhaps most obviously, concern has traditionally been expressed about inward migration into the developed capitalist countries, not outward migration from them. In Britain's case, there was net emigration in most decades of the twentieth century, including the first two decades, the 1960s and the 1970s (Office for National Statistics 2000: 22). As these were the periods which witnessed the erection of major controls, it is clear that the *number* of people migrating inward is not crucial.

Rather it is the national and ethnic origins and the social background of immigrants which has always exercised the immigration controllers. The 'debate' about immigration has always been about 'race' (Sivanandan 1982).

This is hardly a startling new insight. Yet it needs restating and anti-racism has to be the starting point of this chapter. This is not least because the thoroughgoing racism of past British immigration controls has passed without comment or redress by the post-1997 Labour governments. The aim of this chapter, then, is not simply to restate the history of immigration controls in Britain, but to ask a number of questions.

1. Why is racism inseparable from the practice of immigration control? The answer to this must be sought in the historical development of the relation between state and capital and in the ideologies of nationalism and racism that have grown up since the late nineteenth century. This may appear to some to be a needless detour into history and theory, but it is crucial in the context of the debate about whether there can ever be fair or non-racist immigration controls.

2. What is the relationship between the development of immigration controls and the welfare state?

3. What are the prospects for resistance to immigration control at the beginning of the twenty-first century? For some of us, this has always been conceived as a struggle against immigration control as such. The struggle is for a world in which it is not the free trade of commodities for profit which is paramount, but freedom of movement for human beings, without the persecution, racism and suffering which immigration controls bring. Others envisage the construction of 'fair' or 'non-racist' controls as a solution to the harsh treatment of immigrants and asylum seekers which they oppose, and the racism they want an end to. This chapter is a dialogue with those genuine opponents of suffering who take a different view. By contrast, there seems little point in trying to use reasoned argument to persuade ministers like those in Britain's Labour governments since 1997 who have tightened the screw against asylum seekers in particular, while adopting the same old 'firm but fair' rhetoric (for a more detailed critique, see Mynott 2000.) Their actions have increased the persecution of the desperate and desperately poor; they have dragooned more and more public and voluntary sector workers into the position of immigration officers, excluding desperate people from services, and enforcing an apartheid welfare system of vouchers and forced dispersal.

Immigration controls and racism

Despite the widespread acceptance of immigration controls today, migration is central to the human experience. Human beings have moved from one geographical region to another throughout the history of the human race. For the earliest human beings who lived in hunter–gatherer societies, the need to move was constant and the notion of settlement alien. The development first of agricultural, and then of other more advanced forms of production, gave rise to the first settlements and the first states. This did not mean the end of movement by human beings, but it did mean that now movement would become migration across state borders. Moreover, the increasing complexity of social organisation meant that migrations took different forms. Sometimes associated with trade, sometimes with military conquest; sometimes the seeking out of new lands on which to make a living, sometimes the forced migration of slaves captured in ancient wars or traded across the Atlantic. In an important sense, then, movement and migration are constants of human history and fundamental to the human experience.

In this light it is easier to see how historically novel are the systematic immigration controls which were honed by the world's most developed capitalist powers throughout the twentieth century. It is not their novelty, however, which poses problems. Ever since immigration controls were first mooted they have been presented as a simple matter of national interest. This argument alone is decidedly dubious. The very conception of a national interest assumes that different classes within the same territory share the same fundamental interests, despite their disparities of wealth and power and their conflicting experiences of exploitation; but there is another reason for rejecting immigration controls.

Although controls *formally* discriminate on grounds of nationality, racism has fundamentally informed the construction of immigration controls. The ideological justification for control has been a racialised nationalism, and the practice of control by the state has been directed at racialised groups.

If we look at the historical record, it is clear that agitation for the implementation of controls has usually been posed in racist terms or has drawn on racist assumptions. This was certainly the case with the agitation for immigration control in Britain at the beginning of the twentieth century, which eventually led to the 1905 Aliens Act (Foot 1965; Gainer 1972). The intended targets of those who agitated for control were Jewish people. From the 1880s the increasing level of anti-semitism and pogroms led hundreds of thousands to flee westwards to avoid persecution. Between 1875 and 1914, 120 000 Jews settled in Britain – the majority in London's East End but also in cities such as Manchester and Leeds (Foot 1965; Castles and Kosack 1973). It was in this period that the term 'alien' became synonymous with Jew. A racist campaign led by Conservative MPs blamed aliens for overcrowding, criminality, living on 'Poor Relief' and much more. Typical of the speeches made by Conservative MPs was this by Mr Hayes Fisher of Fulham: 'Just as one river could carry a certain amount of sewage, but not the sewage of the whole Kingdom, so one portion of London cannot carry the whole of the pauper and diseased alien immigrants who come into the country' (Foot 1965: 98). Parliamentary speeches were backed by the press, with the *Manchester Evening Chronicle* opposing the right of political asylum as 'sentimental' and wanting an Aliens Bill to exclude 'the dirty, destitute, diseased, verminous and criminal foreigner' (Cohen 1987: 8).

Despite some opposition to its racism, the Aliens Act became law. Its main provisions were to control the entry of 'undesirable aliens' and to deport those who committed a criminal offence or had been in receipt of poor relief. In practice it was Jewish people who were hit by the Act, with cases of denial of entry and refusal of asylum regularly reported in the *Jewish Chronicle*. Thus the first immigration controls introduced in Britain were the result of racist agitation, were racist in their operation and were deliberately directed at working class people.

Nor, in the late nineteenth and early twentieth centuries, was the debate about immigration control and the passage of legislation restricted to Britain. It was in the 1880s and 1890s that restrictions first appeared on Polish labourers in Germany, and in the 1880s on Chinese labourers in the United States (Sassen 1999; Cohen 1991). Such piecemeal controls on particular ethnic and national groups hardened into systematic immigration controls during the first quarter of the twentieth century. Britain's first Aliens Act of 1905 was augmented by further Aliens legislation in 1914 and 1919.

In the United States, language qualifications and quotas were introduced in 1917 and 1921 until the turning point came with the 1924 National Origins (Johnson–Reed) Act of 1924, which is usually seen as effectively closing the United States to transatlantic migration.

In Germany, the original *Gastarbeiter* system was developed and greatly accelerated around the turn of the century. Intensive political management of the labour market allowed German employers to recruit when required from a mainly Slavic external reserve army of labour. The whole process promoted xenophobia and nationalism. It was in 1913, against a background of hostility to Slavic immigration that 'blood-based' citizenship was entrenched in law. Dale cites

Brubaker (1992) in the claim that: 'Citizenship law was framed explicitly to keep the Eastern provinces German by preventing the permanent settlement of "ethnonationally undesired migrants"'. He concludes:

[T]he intertwining of nationalism and racism within the very structure of the labour market was made hard and fast during the late nineteenth century. It was not deliberately planned as a racist strategy of 'divide and rule'. But in practice it was precisely that, and those in power came to realise its potency, and were to consciously apply that knowledge to future immigration policy.

(Dale 1999a: 121)

Above all it was the First World War which acted as a catalyst for the introduction of systematic immigration controls. As Harris has described it:

By the First World War, virtually all the Great Powers were seeking to control movements across their borders. War itself provided a crescendo of hysteria on the issue, sufficient to reverse long-standing commitments and practices relating to the freedom to move. By the 1920s most governments had taken powers to control movement.

(Harris 1996: 6)

Saskia Sassen also locates the First World War as a crucial episode when modern European states strengthened their border-enforcement functions and suddenly started checking passports. She argues that: 'We can see to what extent the contemporary debate about immigration and refugee control is a response to a rather new history for Europe, a history that began with World War One' (Sassen 1999: 77). She suggests that nation states for the first time participated in the identification and regulation of refugees within mass refugee movements: 'The role of the state changed in a fundamental way when the state assumed control over borders and over a growing range of events in its territory' (Sassen 1999: 79). Further, the turn by the United States and Canada in the 1920s to excluding immigrants from entry, had a significant impact on political perceptions within Europe:

It was only when North America closed its borders to immigration which included a disproportionate share of Jewish refugees, that the Western European states experienced the refugee crisis as a crisis, one that affected the interstate system.

(Sassen 1999: 87)

State and capital – 'race' and nation

The First World War was a catalyst in the development of systematic immigration controls because it represented a qualitative shift in the relationship between state and capital and inaugurated a period of greater state intervention into economic and social life. It was never true that capitalism developed as a system of competing capitals quite separate from, but parallel to, a system of competing states. Rather, modern nation states arose in Europe as an integral part of the developing capitalist system. They were, in Marxist terms, superstructures arising on an economic base; but they were superstructures the actions of which fed back into and shaped capitalist development. It is in this sense that the development of capitalism gives rise to modern capitalist nation states, as well as national identities and nationalist movements:

> Any productive capital grows up within the confines of a particular territory, alongside other sibling capitals (they are, as Marx describes them, 'warring brothers'). They are mutually dependent on each other for resources, finance and markets. And they act together to try to shape the social and political conditions in that territory to suit their own purposes.
>
> This involves an effort to 'free' labour from the control of other classes, to remove obstacles to the sales of their products, to create an infrastructure (ports, roads, canals, railways) to fit their requirements, to establish sets of rules for regulating their relations with each other (bourgeois property laws) and to create an armed power which will protect their property both from domestic and external threats. Their efforts to achieve all these things will be aided if they can supplant a mass of dialects and languages with a single form of spoken and written speech. Their aim, in short has to be to create a *national* state power – and with it a national consciousness and language.
>
> (Harman 1991: 9)

In the 'classical' phase of mid-nineteenth century capitalism, that which most closely accorded to the descriptions of Adam Smith's *Wealth of Nations* and in Britain provided the material for Marx's analysis in *Capital*, the role of the state was quite limited. It was certainly more limited than it had been in the preceding centuries or was to become again from the late nineteenth century. By the 1880s, the major capitalist nation states had been formed – by revolution in seventeenth century England and eighteenth century France, by unification in Germany and Italy and by the civil war that created the modern United States. Now a new phase in the development of capitalism took place, famously identified as imperialism by writers as different as the English liberal, John Hobson (1988) and the Russian revolutionary, Lenin (1986). Imperialism should be understood not narrowly as being identified purely with colonialism, but as being characterised by increasing interstate rivalry. This important development within the capitalist system had a significant impact on nationalism. There had been historical moments when nationalist ideologies had been used in struggles against existing forms of oppression. That was the case in the development of capitalist as against absolutist states and it was to be true again in the twentieth century, in the struggle of oppressed nations against the colonising imperialist powers. So, although 'nation', like 'race', is a supra-class category where an imagined commonality overrides conflicting interests based on production, it is necessary to distinguish between nationalism and racism. Racism is premised on the inevitable inferiority of particular groups defined by negatively evaluated characteristics which are assumed to be inherited. As such, unlike nationalism, it has always and everywhere played a reactionary role.

Yet there was across Europe a transformation of nationalisms between 1870 and 1918. Eric Hobsbawm has described this as a move away from the earlier 'Mazzinian' phase in which the old monarchies and aristocracies were contrasted with the 'nation' as 'the body of citizens whose collective sovereignty constituted them a state which was their political expression' (Hobsbawm 1990: 18–19). In its place came a new emphasis on ethnicity and language as the decisive criteria of potential nationhood, and the use of 'race' and 'nation' as interchangeable terms, a development promoted by the rise of scientific racism.

Towards the end of the nineteenth century, therefore, nations could be conceived as natural groups whose cultural symbols were grounded in biological race: 'A racialised nationalism could then conceive of certain "nations" as eternally contaminated, and therefore outside of history' (Miles 1993: 62). In the context of the development of imperialism, it becomes true, as Robert Miles argues, that there is no simple dichotomy between racism and nationalism. Rather: 'the ideologies of racism and nationalism can be interdependent and overlapping . . . so that the boundary of the imagined "nation" is equally a boundary of "race"' (Miles 1993: 79).

What was to become one of the most important expressions of racialised nationalism in the developed capitalist countries in the twentieth century was the entrenchment of immigration controls. Racism was everywhere integral to the development of immigration controls. Particular groups of immigrants were racialised and presented as a threat to the supposedly finite material resources of the receiving nation, as well as its 'culture'. As industrial capitalism led to vast migrations of people both within and, increasingly, across national borders, it created populations drawn from a wider range of national and 'racial' backgrounds. Within the ranks of workers there was the experience of unity in the face of the exploiter, but also the experience of division and competition for scarce resources. In this context, the development of class-based and internationalist forms of organisation and consciousness jostled with the development of a national consciousness and the acceptance of racist ideas.

The post-war picture

If we look at the broad sweep of historical development, it is clear that systematic immigration controls became entrenched during the twentieth century. Yet the manner and determination with which controls were implemented depended on the health of the international capitalist system. In the aftermath of the Second World War, there was a long economic boom in Europe and the United States that lasted until the 1970s. Unprecedented economic expansion saw a massive demand for labour which drove an expansion in migration. Those European countries with colonies and ex-colonies (principally, France, Britain and Holland), looked to them as a source of labour – albeit only after it became apparent that the displaced and the refugees of Europe were not going to be sufficient (Foot 1965; Webber 1991). At the same time, West Germany with its lack of colonies rediscovered the *Gastarbeiter* system. After the movement of millions of ethnic Germans from the East failed to quench the miracle economy's thirst for labour, it turned to Italy, Greece and Turkey recruiting millions more workers (Dale 1999b).

What was happening was that the need of capital for labour power temporarily opened the gates which the nationalism and racism of immigration control would have slammed shut. Opening the gates to migration, however, did not mean that racism disappeared. As Sivanandan has put it: 'What Europe wants is immigrant labour, not the immigrant' (cited in Fekete 1998). The *Gastarbeiter* system, the principles of which animated most European countries' immigration policies, sought to regulate migrant labour, but in the interests of capital and to the detriment of the immigrants. *Gastarbeiter* systems appeared to offer an opportunity to capital to exploit labour power with lower replacement costs and without having to supply the same level of wider social provision that they supplied to workers who were already present. Labour was expected to be flexible and, ideally, disposable. In practice, by the early 1970s settlement and attempts at family reunification were taking place in Belgium, Holland, Germany and France (Webber 1991).

Moreover, there was some tension between the sections of capital most dependent on guestworkers and nation states:

> since large employers in the manufacturing industries wanted a trained and skilled workforce, not a high turnover of unskilled, short term workers. Governments and labour authorities, on the other hand, did not want foreigners to settle and bring their families, and favoured the rotation of temporary, unskilled and rightless workers (Webber 1991: 13).

With the end of the long boom in the 1970s there were about 11 million migrant workers in Europe (Webber 1991: 12). The return of economic crisis led to a shift towards restrictive immigration policies which were accompanied by a rise in racism. Britain had led in this disreputable direction a decade earlier, reforging the link between race and immigration which had been pioneered in the Aliens legislation, but now in the context of black Commonwealth immigration. In part, Britain led the way because its economy had faltered earlier, in the 1960s; in part because the status of Commonwealth immigrants as British citizens gave them legal settlement rights which made it harder to treat them as temporary guests. Of course, once the racist logic of control had been conceded in 1962, it was to be repeated again in the Commonwealth Immigration Act (1968), the Immigration Act (1971), the Nationality Act (1981) and the various asylum Acts of the 1990s.

The final quarter of the twentieth century witnessed the return of periodic recessions, and a drop in the rate of profit which, taken together, can be seen to represent the return of capitalist crisis. It is easier to see now how this has been a period marked by the political project now known as neo-liberalism. This has sought to open up as many areas of the economy as possible to the free market and break from the social democratic consensus of mixed economy and public welfare which characterised the long post-war boom. Yet we must remember that this is precisely a political project rather than an inevitable process going under the name of 'globalisation' – which is so often a prescription masquerading as a description. (For a full discussion of globalisation see Held *et al.* 1999.) It is true that there has been a growth in international trade, flows of finance capital and to a certain extent cross-border production and ownership. What is crucial, however, is that neo-liberalism is not seeking to abolish nation states, but to reconfigure the relationship between state and capital. It is an attempt by the strongest capitalist states, in particular, to offload the economic and social costs of crisis.

But it leaves a gaping contradiction in the ideology and the practice of governments: 'Freedom of movement, defended as a right for capital, is seen as a privilege for labour' (Dale 1999b: 4). This contradiction has been exacerbated since the collapse of the 'communist' regimes of eastern Europe and the former Soviet Union. As Gary Younge has argued:

> Our governments are trapped in a morally warped and ideologically unsustainable paradigm. They applaud the free movement of capital; they abhor the free movement of labour.
>
> (Younge 2001)

The construction of a 'Fortress Europe', which was identified by critics over a decade ago (Gordon 1989; Cohen 1991), continued apace throughout the 1990s. The project of the European Union was to create free movement of labour within its boundaries while strengthening border controls at the boundaries. Immigration controls have been harmonised in the sense that they have been constructed and tightened where they were previously weak or nonexistent. In Spain and Italy the more *laissez faire* attitude to 'illegals' came under pressure in the 1980s and 1990s, leading to stricter immigration controls (Fekete 1998). There has also been a harmonisation of policies in relation to asylum seekers and welfare provision.

It is not true, then, that a new era of globalisation with its growing international linkages is breaking down the power of nation states and provides the prospect of undermining regimes of immigration control, which appears to be the source of Nigel Harris's 'cautious optimism' (Harris 1996). Both the European Union and the United States have relentlessly strengthened immigration controls over the past two decades. In western Europe, the process of racialisation of particular groups of immigrants which was pioneered in the late nineteenth century and reforged in relation to black and third world peoples during the long boom, is occurring anew with refugees and asylum seekers as its core subjects.

Today, the 'immigrants' who are problematised are still those who are working class or poor and whose 'culture' ('race' being a rather discredited concept) is presented as different. They are still invariably presented as a threat to the limited material resources of the nation, despite the exploitation they face, and the extensive evidence that immigrants are net contributors to the economy of the country they arrive in and do not take jobs which would otherwise go to existing residents (Harris 1995: 186–213; Glover *et al.* 2001). The supposed threat they pose can then be used to justify not only their exclusion from the country, but their exclusion from welfare provision. However, because of the racist assumptions which accompany immigration controls, exclusion can affect not only those people who lack the required immigration status, but by extension those who are assumed to be ineligible or undeserving because their 'culture' (for which, read 'race') puts them outside of the genuine nation.

The political effect of immigration control is then twofold. It institutionalises racism, but it is also part of the attempt to encourage the majority of people, especially working class people, to identify themselves in nationalistic or racial terms, rather than in terms of class. This attempt has always been met with resistance, but in so far as it is successful it encourages workers to identify with their 'own' state and all the classes within it. The solution to social problems can then be posed in terms of national or racial unity in the battle over scarce resources, rather than in terms of working class unity to challenge the existing distribution of resources and the priorities of capitalist economies. Immigration controls are thus racist *and* against the class interests of workers.

Immigration controls and welfare

Immigration controls are by their nature exclusionary, but they can operate both externally and internally. External controls consist, in the main, of border controls. This physical control of borders is what most people associate with immigration control. Physical control is enforced by high walls and barbed wire fences, by the familiar passport checks and, increasingly, by the use of sniffer dogs and carbon monoxide detectors to hunt out migrants stowed clandestinely on vehicles. Border controls have increasingly been augmented over recent years by pre-entry controls – carrier liability laws which fine airlines, rail companies and shipping lines for carrying inadequately documented passengers, and the imposition of visa restrictions on particular countries.

By contrast, internal controls consist, at their most basic, of identity checks inside the territory of the nation state. Checking on immigration status can discover whether an individual has gained the permission of the state to enter and remain, thus putting clandestine immigrants at risk of imprisonment or deportation. However, checks on immigration status by employers and officials of all kinds are also a means to enforce restrictions on the right to work or receive support services on the part of all 'persons subject to immigration control', thus exerting a powerful discipline on them.

The link between immigration control and access to welfare has been a feature of immigration controls in Britain since the Aliens Acts (see Chapter 3). An 'undesirable alien' was defined as 'someone who cannot show that he has in his possession or is in a position to obtain the means of supporting himself and his dependants' or who 'owing to any disease or infirmity appears likely to become a charge on the rates or otherwise a detriment to the public' (Cohen 1987: 21). This obsessive fear that immigrants will claim public funds, and attempts to prevent them doing so, are mirrored in the immigration controls of other European countries and the United States (Cohen 1991). In the 1980s and 1990s harmonisation of reception policies for asylum seekers across the European Union (Bank 2000) has made the deliberate social exclusion of asylum seekers the cutting edge of governments' long-established obsession with preventing immigrants' access to welfare.

However, there is an important difference between the past and present. The imposition of systematic immigration controls with their prohibitions on access to welfare took place in the early twentieth century when the first elements of the social democratic welfare state were being laid down. In such conditions it was easier for the state – sometimes supported by the labour movement – to argue that a genuine social contract was being forged between capital and labour. In return for workers adopting a nationalistic loyalty to 'their' state (preferably with a social democratic government in office), in place of internationalist class solidarity which united immigrant with non-immigrant, the state would provide a degree of welfare provision which had not existed before under *laissez faire* capitalism.

But the turn towards a greater linkage between control and welfare in the late 1970s and early 1980s, which in Britain hit black people hardest (Gordon 1985; Gordon and Newnham 1985), coincided with the beginnings of the Thatcherite attack on the welfare state; and today, the systematic exclusion of 'persons subject to immigration control' and the creation of apartheid welfare provision for asylum seekers takes place in the context of an unprecedented neo-liberal onslaught on the welfare state. This makes it more difficult for those forces who want to present the removal of rights from minorities such as asylum seekers as the price for defending or extending general welfare provision for a mainstream majority. This is simply because the onslaught on the minority is happening at the same time as the erosion of provision for the majority. This is not to claim that racist arguments are not being put or will disappear – quite the reverse, they are likely to remain a constant feature of official politics and the news media. It is rather to claim that the worsening of material conditions for the majority creates a lived experience which can be appealed to and out of which an alternative to racism can be constructed by those seeking to stress a unity of interest between migrants and non-migrants.

What does all of this mean for those of us who wish to defend welfare provision in general and challenge the particular restrictions imposed on asylum seekers and other migrants subject to immigration control?

The state provision of welfare is a gain which has been won by progressive social movements of the past – even if alternative models of 'popular welfare' may have been envisaged by some as a better alternative than 'state welfare' (Jones and Novak 2000). The problem is that the welfare state as it developed in the first half of the twentieth century (and was then massively extended after 1945) represented a compromise between the interests of capital and the needs of working class people. One feature of the compromise was its national basis. The welfare state was constructed, ironically enough, as a mechanism to make nationally organised capital more efficient in its competition and rivalry with other nationally organised capitalisms. Hence the nationalism which was built into welfare provision from an early stage – such as the restrictions on eligibility for state pensions before the First World War (Cohen 1996). At its best, the post-war social democratic settlement did move a long way beyond the social imperialist origins of welfare provision and was based on genuine co-operative and caring principles. Witness Bevan's original belief that the National Health Service should be free to all who needed it. Sadly, that was the exception in the development of British welfare.

So the provision of services through the welfare state was a contradictory phenomenon. On the one hand, it represented a beachhead for caring and co-operation against the cut-throat competition and rivalry which characterise capitalism. On the other, it could often exhibit a bureaucratic and sometimes moralistic approach to planning, in the style of the state-directed command economy, rather than a version of planning which grows out of genuine democratic discussion of popular needs and priorities. Hence the legitimate criticisms which arose from the left in the 1960s and 1970s (London Edinburgh Weekend Return Group 1980).

In practice, however, it was not the criticisms from the left, but right wing neo-liberalism which informed the changes to the welfare state which were unleashed in the 1980s and 1990s. In Britain, the

Thatcherite project led the way and now the New Labour approach to welfare has continued with even more of the same – to the extent that we are going beyond cut-backs to the removal of most of the central planks of the British welfare state. There are increasing restrictions on the claiming of social security benefits under the welfare to work scheme. There has been a huge transfer of public housing out of local authority control, with an ambition to transfer all of it within a decade. There has been a deliberate decision to promote private pension provision while letting the basic state pension wither on the vine. There has been a removal of free access to higher education and a steady move towards selection and away from the comprehensive model in state education. After the terrible neglect of infrastructure, especially capital spending, the Conservatives' Private Finance Initiative has been taken up and applied much more widely by Labour than its inventors could have imagined.

Britain and the United States may be further along the road than other European countries, but the direction across the world is the same. Just as capital is reorganising industry away from state ownership and maximising the penetration of free market mechanisms, nation states are radically reshaping the post-war welfare settlement on neo-liberal principles.

Under these conditions, it is necessary to defend such existing welfare provision as benefits working class and poor people. This would include council housing and comprehensive education, for example. It also means arguing for the reversal of measures such as the de-coupling of the level of the state pension from that of average earnings. At the same time it is necessary to argue for, and as far as possible create, forms of public provision which are really accountable and designed to meet the needs of the users of services, rather than treating individuals as units of labour power, viewed fundamentally in terms of their utility to capital.

This would mean no return to past examples of enforced uniformity which sometimes marked the classic social democratic welfare state. Such an approach was rooted (at least in part) in a condescending attitude which saw reformers as doing things *for* working class people who were not capable of running society themselves. It would mean no return to the model of the family as a male breadwinner with a dependent wife and children.

It would also mean, crucially for our purposes, a break from the fundamental nationalism at the heart of welfare provision under capitalism. The capitalist state has always seen its job as securing the interests of nationally based capital. Any new forms of social provision would have to treat people according to their needs as human beings, not according to their national origins or formal citizenship. Part of the struggle to create such welfare provision would be the reintegration of asylum seekers and those subject to immigration control into existing welfare provision.

To pose this as what we need to fight for is to go against the stream of neo-liberalism across Europe and the United States. But it also goes beyond a criticism of the dominant policy of capital to implicitly challenge *capitalism*. That is a big challenge, but it is one which is being taken up by a new movement whose adherents are generalising from the many specific issues which concern them, to see global capitalism as the overarching problem. In this sense, the situation for those who wish to resist immigration controls and their effects is more heartening than for many years. While nation states have been building their fortresses and transnational capital has proclaimed the benefits to all of globalisation, a new anti-capitalist mood and movement have developed in the heartlands of European and North American capitalism.

Prospects for resistance: from anti-racism to anti-capitalism

Since the demonstrations that caused the collapse of the World Trade Organisation ministerial meeting at the end of November 1999, there has crystallised in the advanced capitalist countries a politically active minority that sees global capitalism as the source of the world's ills. It is this sense of totality, of the system itself being at fault that distinguishes this new anti-capitalist movement from campaigns that focus on specific issues and grievances.

(Callinicos 2001)

The appearance of anti-capitalism should be hugely heartening to those who share the kind of outlook on immigration controls, racism and welfare articulated in this chapter. There are so many reasons for this: its success in pushing the powerful onto the defensive, at least intellectually, after a decade in which neo-liberalism has been rampant; its self-consciously international outlook which means that the rights of asylum seekers are raised – for instance, as part of the call for a 'social Europe' in the protests at the intergovernmental meetings in Nice at the end of 2000. Not least is the way that the high profile of the movement reaches beyond its active participants to influence other struggles which do not formally come under its umbrella. John Rees has argued:

In this sense anti-capitalist movements are giving a particular colouration to every other movement of resistance against the system, no matter how partial. Campaigners against tube privatisation in London suddenly see Balfour Beatty, the likely beneficiaries, in the light of the campaign to stop the building of the Ilisu dam in Turkey by the same company. Trade unionists are now being thrust into a politicised world where environmental protesters and socialists are their allies, where the effects of imperialism and global capitalism on the Third World are being raised point blank, and where mass action is increasingly being seen as the accepted method of struggle.

(Rees 2001: 7)

A further instance could be given – that of the campaigns to defend asylum seekers which have taken off in Britain in response to the voucher schemes, forced dispersal and increased detention ushered in by the Immigration and Asylum Act (1999). So bad is the treatment of asylum seekers by the Labour government that new organisations and layers of individuals, especially from the voluntary sector, have been drawn into activity alongside the more established anti-racist organisations. In some areas, churchgoers have begun to try to set up arrangements to swap vouchers for cash, thus trying to undermine the voucher system, quite independently of established political activists. In this climate, it has become easier than ever to highlight the hypocrisy of governments and corporations which champion free movement of capital as a vital necessity for the world, while they treat free movement of people as a heresy. An observation long commonplace on the Marxist left is now shared by much wider numbers, pushed into wider consciousness by the juxtaposition of neo-liberal exhortations of the need for globalisation with the demonisation of migrants.

This is a situation where people can move from a strongly felt liberal humanitarianism to a radical questioning of global capitalism very quickly. They can be persuaded by arguments, such as those in this chapter, which have their roots in much longer histories – whether of the workers movement, the anti-racist movement or black people's experiences over a generation or more.

The strategic challenge, therefore, is to bring about a creative fusion between anti-racism and anti-capitalism. Our challenge is to encourage an interaction in practical campaigning and in theoretical debate. This fusion can draw on the enthusiasm, dynamism and often detailed knowledge of specific issues present in the new movement, and combine it with the experiences and insights of an older generation of activists, strengthening and revitalising both in the process. There is one other thing that the fusion of anti-racism and anti-capitalism can do.

It can encourage the already-existing international outlook of the anti-capitalist movement to become a consistent internationalism, embracing an anti-imperialist and anti-racist perspective. An understanding can be generated of how racism originated in the transatlantic slave trade and classical imperialism, and is perpetuated by the operation of global capitalism today. How the workings of global capital – imperialism in its modern incarnation – have created the conditions which led to the forced migration of millions across the third world; and how the immigration controls of Fortress Europe and of the West as a whole seek to damn the flow of people when it does not want to exploit them.

An anti-capitalist movement can be built with anti-racism at its heart, a movement which fights for unity across the borders of nationality and 'race'.

Just as capitalist development is global, shaping the patterns and motivation of different migrations, so the response to it must be internationalist – insisting that the forces to challenge it exist in every country and on every continent. To create a world order which is truly committed to the welfare of the world's people, the freedom to move must be among the freedoms we fight for.

References

Bank, R. (2000) 'Europeanising the reception of asylum seekers: The opposite of welfare state politics' in Bommes, M. and Geddes, A. (eds) *Welfare and Immigration: challenging the borders of the welfare state*, London: Routledge, pp 148–169.

Brubaker, W. (1992) *Citizenship and Nationhood in France and Germany*, Cambridge: Harvard.

Callinicos, A (2001) *The Anti-Capitalist Movement and the Revolutionary Left*, London: Socialist Workers Party.

Castles, S. and Kosack, G. (1973) *Immigrant Workers and Class Structure in Western Europe*, London: Oxford University Press for the Institute of Race Relations.

Castles, S. and Miller, M.J. (1998) *The Age of Migration: international population movements in the modern world* (2nd edn), Basingstoke: Macmillan.

Cohen, S. (1987) *It's the Same Old Story*. Manchester: Manchester City Council.

——(1991) *Imagine There's No Countries: 1992 and international immigration controls against migrants, immigrants and refugees*. Manchester: Greater Manchester Immigration Aid Unit.

—— (1996) 'Anti-semitism, immigration controls and the welfare state', in D.Taylor (ed.), *Critical Social Policy: a reader*, London: Sage, pp 27–47.

Dale, G. (1999a) 'Germany: nation and immigration' in Dale, G. and Cole, M. (eds) *The European Union and Migrant Labour*, Oxford: Berg, pp 113–146.

—— (1999b) 'Introduction' in Dale, G. and Cole, M. (eds) *The European Union and Migrant Labour*, Oxford: Berg, pp 1–14.

Fekete, L. (1998) 'Blackening the economy: the path to convergence' *Race and Class*, 39(4): 1–22.

Foot, P. (1965) *Immigration and Race in British Politics*, Harmondsworth: Penguin.

Ford, R. (1994) 'Current and future migration flows' in Spencer, S. (ed.) *Strangers and Citizens: a positive approach to migrants and refugees*, London: Rivers Oram Press, pp 44–90.

Gainer, B. (1972) *The Alien Invasion: the origins of the Aliens Act of 1905*, London: Heinemann

Glover, S., Gott, C., Loizillon, A., Portes, J., Price, R., Spencer, S., Srinivasan, V. and Willis, C., (2001) *Migration: an economic and social analysis, Research Development and Statistics Directorate Occasional Paper No. 67*, London: Home Office.

Gordon, P. (1985) *Policing Immigration: Britain's internal controls*, London: Pluto Press.

—— (1989) *Fortress Europe? The meaning of 1992*, London: Runnymede Trust.

Gordon, P. and Newnham, A. (1985) *Passport to Benefits? Racism in social security*, London: Child Poverty Action Group and Runnymede Trust.

Harman, C. (1991) 'The state and capitalism today', *International Socialism*, 51, Summer: 3–54.

Harris, N. (1996) *The New Untouchables: immigration and the new world worker*, London: Penguin

Held, D., McGrew, A., Goldblatt, D. and Perraton, J. (1999) *Global Transformations: politics, economics and culture*, Cambridge: Polity Press.

Hobsbawm, E. (1990) *Nations and Nationalism since 1780: programme, myth, reality*, Cambridge: Cambridge University Press.

Hobson, J.A. (1988) *Imperialism: a study* (3rd edn; originally 1905), London: Unwin Hyman.

Jones, C. and Novak, T. (2000) 'Class struggle, self help and popular welfare' in Lavalette, M and Mooney, G., *Class Struggle and Social Welfare*, London: Routledge.

Lenin, V. I. (1986) *Imperialism, the Highest Stage of Capitalism: a popular out-line* (originally 1916), Moscow: Progress Publishers.

London Edinburgh Weekend Return Group (1980) *In and Against the State*, London: Pluto Press.

Miles, R. (1993) *Racism after 'Race' Relations*, London: Routledge.

Mynott, E (2000) 'Analysing the creation of apartheid for asylum seekers in the UK', *Community, Work and Family*, 3(3): 311–331.

Office for National Statistics (2000) *Social Trends 30: 2000 Edition*, London: The Stationery Office.

Rees, J. (2001) 'Anti-capitalism, reformism and socialism', *International Socialism*, 90, Spring: 3–40.

Sassen, S. (1999) *Guests and Aliens*, New York: The New Press.

Sivanandan, A. (1982) *A Different Hunger: writings on black resistance*, London: Pluto Press.

Stalker, P. (2000) *Workers Without Frontiers: the impact of globalization on international migration*, London: Lynne Rienner/International Labour Office.

Webber, F. (1991) 'From ethnocentrism to Euro-racism', *Race and Class*, 32(3): 11–17.

Younge, G. (2001) 'Penalising the Poor', *Guardian*, 19 March.

3 From aliens to asylum seekers

A history of immigration controls and welfare in Britain

Debra Hayes

This chapter intends to examine the origins of the connection between immigration status and welfare entitlement, and to explore how this has developed through the twentieth century. At the start of the new millennium we have reached a point where: 'In Western Europe, refugees have begun to look like beggars at the gate, or even thieves' (Harding 2000: 10). Focusing on the 1905 Aliens Act, the first attempt to control entry into the UK, and the debates which preceded it, illustrates a long-term construction of the refugee in such a way, as burdensome, needy, socially costly, and consequently undesirable. What I hope to show is how this logic, which constructs the 'outsider' as costly (financially, socially and morally), has not only been used to control entry, but has twinned with a further powerful ideology concerning welfare and nation, producing immigration controls which consistently place at their centre the need to access welfare as grounds for refusal of entry, and a welfare state which ensures provision is restricted to 'its own'.

The lobby for control

In 1870s Victorian Britain concern began to be expressed about the number of aliens arriving. The 'refugee question' entered public debate both in newspapers and parliament, fear and panic being its overwhelming features (Gainer 1972; Garrard 1971). It was Russian and Polish immigration which became central, as Jews fled pogroms and widespread persecution in Eastern Europe. A Select Committee was appointed in 1888 to:

> Inquire into the laws existing in the United States and elsewhere on the subject of the immigration of destitute aliens, and as to the

extent and effect of such immigration into the UK, and to report whether it is desirable to impose any, and if so, what restrictions on such immigration.

(Select Committee 1889a: i)

The issue of control was on the agenda, but it was not simply a question of numbers. It was the poor eastern European Jew who was to become the focus for control and in the run up to the first piece of immigration control in 1905, 'alien' became synonymous with 'Jew'. The Select Committee contributed to this process by focusing much attention on the habits and lifestyle of this group, as opposed to Scandinavians arriving in large numbers at Hull, as 'these immigrants are of a respectable class' (Select Committee 188b9: v). How far these Jewish aliens were a burden on the rates, became a point for discussion at the Committee. Nevertheless, the Committee fell short of calling for controls and with respect to aliens felt, 'the fears and complaints which have been expressed concerning their effect upon our own population will appear exaggerated' (Select Committee 1889b: vii).

Try, try and try again

Nevertheless, the lobby gained momentum and there were failed attempts to introduce a Bill into Parliament in 1894, 1898 and 1904, before the Aliens Act was finally passed in 1905 (Ford and Ford 1957; Hansard 1901–1905). By the time a Royal Commission was established to report in 1903, the terms of reference were clear, its purpose, 'to enquire into the character and extent of the evils which are attributed to the unrestricted immigration of aliens' (Royal Commission 1903a Vol. i: 5). The kind of features attributed to aliens were that they were, impoverished, destitute, deficient in cleanliness, liable to introduce infectious diseases, criminals, anarchists, prostitutes, caused overcrowding and raised rents (Royal Commission 1903a Vol. i: 5). The Royal Commission heard from many 'experts' with a great deal to say on the alien question, much of which was a matter of personal opinion. It seemed that before the advent of the alien, working class life was free of hardship. Taking evidence from Mrs Ayres, a midwife, the Royal Commission was told:

It used to be a street occupied by poor English and Irish people. In the afternoons you would see the steps inside cleaned, and the women with their clean white aprons sat in summer times inside the doors, perhaps at needlework, with their little children about them.

Now it is a seething mass of refuse and filth . . . the stench is disgraceful . . . They are such an unpleasant, indecent people.

(cited in Garrard 1971: 51)

In the Houses of Parliament, the Tories of the day became unusually concerned about the condition of the English working class, Major Evans-Gordon lamenting: 'Not a day passes but English families are ruthlessly turned out to make room for these foreign invaders' (Hansard 1902 Vol. 101: 1273).

In a similar vein, Cathcart Wilson implored:

What was the use of spending thousands of pounds in building beautiful workmen's dwellings if the places of our workpeople, the backbone of the country, were to be taken by the refuse and scum of foreign Nations?

(Hansard 1903 Vol. 118: 137)

As Jewish refugees became responsible for the social problems of the period, attention focused now on their likely social cost. Sir Howard Vincent, a vocal anti-alien argued:

These alien immigrants were in such a condition that they had to be relieved by the Jewish Board of Guardians . . . and 2,015, including 1,100 Russians and Poles, had to be supported by the poor rates of London.

(Hansard 1901 Vol. 195: 1208)

As the Royal Commission began to construct how the machinery of control might operate, the question of 'means' became key. Immigration officers would need to form judgements about who was likely to be a burden on the rates. In fact, the bulk of relief given to aliens was medical relief, not money, and was provided by Jewish charities (Royal Commission 1903a Vol. i: 16); but establishing that *all* aliens were burdensome on the rates was necessary in the ideological battle to secure controls.

Disease and deviance

There are two further features of the demonising of Jewish refugees taking place in this period which are worthy of mention, and which, like much of the mythology, share striking similarities with current discourses. These are the linking of the Jew with both crime and disease. These processes served to strengthen the calls for controls at the point of entry, as well as establishing that Jews were undeserving of help if resident. Crime figures were used regularly in Parliamentary debates to show aliens were more criminally motivated than the native population. Fifteen per cent of prisoners tried in north London in 1901 were said to be foreigners (Hansard 1902 Vol. 102: 30). The picture was of increasing crime in London, for which the alien was to blame. In addition, the Royal Commission focused a great deal of attention on the question of health and disease. This was despite evidence from medical officers, such as Dr Herbert Williams, who concluded:

As to their health, I should say it was fairly good. The number of cases of infectious disease introduced that I have detected amongst these people has not been numerous speaking as a whole. I cannot say that much infectious disease has come into this country among these people.

(Royal Commission 1903b Vol. ii: 6113)

Despite an array of evidence from medical officers from London, Liverpool and Manchester concerning lower infant mortality rates, lower death rates, lower rates of alcoholism, higher levels of breast feeding and better diet among the Jewish population than the native working class (Royal Commission 1903b Vol. ii: 21742–21799), the linking of the alien Jew with disease in the popular mind had already taken place.

Visions of plague-bearing aliens were reinforced by terrifying fantasies of contagious diseases carried by garments often made up in rooms where children were lying ill with smallpox, scarlet fever and other maladies.

(Gainer 1972: 128)

Anti-aliens in Parliament would return to these images regularly, in their calls for the first controls. Major Evans-Gordon again:

Smallpox and scarlet fever have unquestionably been introduced by aliens . . . and trachoma, a contagious disease, which is the third principal cause of total loss of sight, and favus, a disgusting and contagious disease of the skin, have been and are being introduced by these aliens.

(Hansard 1905 Vol. 145: 711)

The imagery was often of contamination from aliens who 'introduce the plague' (Hansard 1901 Vol. 93: 1317), who bring 'danger of epidemic disease' (Hansard 1903 Vol. 118: 944) and who are referred to as 'sewage' (Hansard 1905 Vol. 145: 754) or 'scum' (Hansard 1904 Vol. 133: 1077) or 'deleterious and objectionable matter' (Hansard 1904 Vol. 133: 1084).

We can see how, before the introduction of immigration controls, a very powerful image had been established in the popular mind, which saw the Jewish refugee as inherently problematic. At the same time as being needy, socially costly, poor and burdensome, they were also less deserving of help because of their association with crime, dirt and disease. These images played a part in establishing the first controls, but also as we shall see, have continued to dominate discourses around immigrants, asylum seekers and refugees since.

The 1905 Aliens Act

The 1905 Aliens Act only applied to steerage passengers – 'undesirables' it seems were unlikely to travel in first or second class. Those to be rejected fell into four main categories of undesirability: the diseased, the insane, the criminal and those thought likely to be a burden on the public purse.

An 'undesirable immigrant' was someone who, inter alia, either (a) cannot show that he has in his possession or is in a position to obtain the means of supporting himself and his dependants or (b) owing to any disease or infirmity appears likely to become a charge on the rates or otherwise a detriment to the public. In other words English welfare was to be denied to the foreign sick and the foreign poor.

(1905 Aliens Act cited in Cohen 1996: 80)

A new body of officials was created, immigration officers, who would work at ports of entry alongside medical inspectors. Their duties were concerned with interviewing bewildered arrivals, asking them to empty their pockets and judging whether they fell into any of the four categories above. In the first year of the Act's operation, of nearly 28,000 inspected, 935 were refused, the vast majority of these (733) on the grounds of insufficient means (HM Inspector of Aliens 1906: 767). In short, the vast majority were rejected because they could not prove they could support themselves without some help. This pattern continued, and whilst the number inspected reduced dramatically, to around 11,000 in 1910, the number of refusals remained constant at just over a thousand in 1910, 837 of which were on the grounds of insufficient means (HM Inspector of Aliens 1910). In a short number of years then, the proportion of refusals in relation to the number inspected, had risen dramatically, and the question of means remained central. The *Jewish Chronicle* newspaper is a very important source of information about the early workings of the Act as it commented weekly on the rejections and on the appeals which had taken place. As the newly formed Appeal Boards exercised their powers, the newspaper noted their inconsistency. These boards were set up 'as and when' necessary each week, geographically close to ports of entry. They heard the cases, kept little in the way of formal records and interpreted whether the Act had been operated correctly. Appellants had some opportunity to call witnesses or supporters, but as many of these were in other UK cities, this was not always possible. The use of interpreters was also haphazard. An editorial entitled 'Aliens at Grimsby' illustrates the confusion in the use of the financial 'means test'. This £5 test seems to have become the only way to test economic viability, a hard and fast rule, rather than a guide (*Jewish Chronicle* 1906f). Without the £5 in the pocket, it was assumed they were going to be burdensome, whatever their skills or indeed whatever they were fleeing.

Fit for Britain?

The other main category of rejections, those on health grounds, are difficult to disentangle from the question of means. This is because health and poor health were constructed in such a way as to differentiate between those who could make a viable economic contribution to Britain and those who may be a burden on the rates. Medical rejections were often quite vague, reflecting as much a concern with productivity without recourse to the public purse, as the threat of disease. These were reported in the *Jewish Chronicle* and included such cases as: a 9-year-old girl, rejected because she was 'deaf and dumb' (1906a); 37-year-old Rosa Presler, declared to be suffering from 'weakness' (1906b); David Kuperberg whose wife had been killed in a pogrom, rejected because he was aged 50 (1906c); a Warsaw tailor, Wolf Relasky, aged 47, rejected on grounds of heart disease (1906d); Gitel Sholk, aged 22, rejected on grounds of being 'dwarfed and deformed' (1906d); Jacob Liebman, a butcher aged 45, rejected as 'suffering from a dilated heart and senility' (1907b). The case of Lieb Kopelow and his family illustrates how arguments about means and health converged. The family won their appeal after original rejections on medical grounds once the Board were: 'Satisfied that it was a good case as the people are in comfortable middle class circumstances and in no way liable to become chargeable to others for their maintenance' (1906e). Editorial comments in the newspaper illustrated the farcical nature of the interpretation of the Act.

> On Friday last three appeal cases were heard at Great Tower Street. In the first a man was refused admission apparently for no other reason than that he was suffering from a hernia. Surely it cannot be contended that this is 'a disease or infirmity which is likely to cause the sufferer to become a charge upon the rates or otherwise a detriment to the public'. Thousands of persons having hernia are useful citizens – they wear trusses.
>
> (*Jewish Chronicle* 1907a)

As other commentators have noted (Cohen 1996), such determinations are a direct forerunner to the present-day use of immigration rules, which prevent entry to anyone who may have 'recourse to public funds'. Of great significance also was the framework set up following the 1905 Act to establish 'internal' immigration controls. In fact, the Act included the provision to deport aliens should they be convicted of a criminal offence, or if they were found to have been in receipt of parochial relief within a year of residence. Cohen (1996: 81) notes that over a thousand people were deported in the first four years of the Act. We can see how in the initial operation of the first piece of legislation to control aliens, access to public money remains key, both at the point of entry and internally.

Nation, Empire and welfare

The context within which the debates around the aliens question took place is of importance in understanding the relationship between welfare and immigration control. As the British Empire flourished in the nineteenth century the role of biological science gained prominence, on the back of Darwin's ideas about natural selection. Increasingly complex biological classifications gave a pseudo-scientific veneer to the theory of 'race'.

> From this time 'race' increasingly came to refer to a biological type of human being, and science purported to demonstrate not only the number and characteristics of each 'race', but also a hierarchical relationship between them.
>
> (Miles 1989: 32)

By the end of the nineteenth century, then, the idea was firmly established that races were different and unequal. The newly emerging 'science' of eugenics could now argue that certain 'races' were of 'poor stock' and not good for the future prospects of the Empire (see Semmell 1960; Searle 1971). Whilst it was taken for granted that the British were morally, intellectually and physically superior to much of the globe, the Empire was to be jolted by near defeat in the Boer War, when the real state of the British working class was to be exposed. In fact, the whole thrust towards the development of welfare came from this panic about Britain's declining dominance on the world stage. So the very same ideology which demanded immigration control – maintaining and improving the nation and its stock – provided the thrust for the first welfare reforms of the twentieth century (see Williams 1989, 1996; Cohen 1996; Hayes 2000). As Germany and the United States began to grab their share of the world markets, Britain experienced panic. What had been irrefutable global dominance now looked insecure. Under the banner of 'national efficiency', concern shifted to the health of the nation, for how could the nation dominate if its populace were not fit for work or war? Here the influence of Darwinism could be seen, as 'social Darwinism' gained acceptance. Attention focused on those not fit for the nation as such leading figures as Karl Pearson called for controls on reproduction among the 'unfit', as well as the barring of undesirable aliens (Cohen 1996: 32). Welfare reform became central to building this nation and of course, the welfare of its own people must take precedence over others. The great Liberal reform programme of 1906–1914, which included the 1908 Old Age Pensions Act and the 1911 National Insurance Act, in reality 'emphasised the necessity for breeding an Imperial race in Great Britain if the Empire were to remain both British and strong' (Semmell 1960: 28). Early social reformers, in particular the Fabians, were heavily influenced by eugenics. The Webbs, George Bernard Shaw, Marie Stopes and others believed that science could build up strong parts of the nation, and eliminate the weak. Marie Stopes' motivation in developing contraception was to 'reduce the numbers of the burgeoning lumpenproletariat'.

> Non-Britons came even lower on the Darwinian pecking order. In those times it was the Jews who were regarded as posing the chief threat of alien dilution of English blood. Bernard Shaw described the Jews as 'the real enemy, the invader from the East, the ruffian, the oriental parasite'.
>
> (*Guardian* 1997: 2)

Not only was the climate conducive to winning the argument about immigration control, as witnessed by the passing of the 1905 Act, but in the emerging welfare state of the twentieth century, the limits had to be set; welfare is for our own.

Exclusive welfare

As we have seen, welfare has never been universal, but has at its heart the premise of exclusion. Exclusion of the unfit and undeserving and exclusion of those considered outside of nation. The two key pieces of legislation in the Liberal reforming Government from 1906, the 1908 Old Age Pensions Act and the 1911 National Insurance Act, contained both residency and citizenship requirements (Cohen 1996: 82–83). There were ongoing concerns about aliens accessing 'out-of-work' donations, which were not extended to them, and the Ministry of Labour sent secret instructions to Labour Exchanges for unemployed black seamen to be kept ignorant of their right to the donation (Williams 1989: 158).

So, what of the golden age of welfare, the establishment of the welfare state in the aftermath of the Second World War? Surely now welfare was to be universal, a matter of right for all citizens? It was in precisely this period that we saw the first significant black immigration into the UK, and it is now pertinent to ask the question: were these gains to be extended to those immigrants, who after all, were not 'aliens', but British citizens? The unfortunate truth is that these newcomers were constructed very much as migrant workers and not as citizens with full rights of access to that emerging welfare. So, black citizens were simply not considered in the massive housing reform programme of the post-war Labour Government (Jacobs 1985; Ginsburg 1988/9). Responsibility for the black arrivals in the 1950s was left to the private market – with well-documented consequences. It was some time before black families were to enter the council house sector and then they waited longer for the worst tenancies (Ginsburg 1988/9). Like Jewish refugees before them, they were then to be blamed for the housing problems where they were forced to reside.

> Immigrants have somehow interrupted and destroyed an earlier Golden Age . . . the immigrant becomes the scapegoat for a number of social problems which existed before he came, and whose intensity is not decreased by preventing his entry.
>
> (Garrard 1971: 5)

In the 1960s, as black families chose to stay or found it impossible to return, 'assimilation' became the dominant discourse. Education was then to become the most significant arm of the welfare state responsible for controlling the black population (Carby 1982). A period of intense lobbying was to ensue around the evils of immigration, not dissimilar to that described up to the passing of the 1905 Aliens Act (Foot 1965). As the question of numbers became central, black people were problematised by their very presence. Carby describes how this translated at school level, with concerns about the *proportion* of black children in classes. This resulted in 'bussing' pupils out of particular schools and requests for passports in particular London Education Authorities before children could be put on school registers (Gordon and Newnham 1985: 68).

Disease re-emerges

As we have seen previously, disease and ill health were grounds for refusal of entry from the beginning of immigration controls. Debates about control re-emerged in relation to black immigrants from the 1950s and again the threat to the physical and moral health of the nation became a common theme. Images and distortions about disease were used to gain further restrictions. The medical establishment was a powerful lobby in calls for more controls on black entry. In the 1950s and 1960s panic was expressed about the incidence of turberculosis (TB) among the immigrant population (Ahmad 1993). Despite its long presence in the UK, TB came to be seen as a disease brought in from the outside. Calls for compulsory screening of immigrants in this period exaggerated the risks and strengthened the calls for more and more controls. Pulmonary TB remains a disease which will normally result in refusal of entry clearance. Linking particular racial groups with particular disease has been most obviously evidenced through racist discourses around HIV/AIDS. Whilst evidence of the virus is not grounds for refusal of entry into the UK, this linkage reinforces the connection between 'immigrants' and undesirability. Refusal of entry on health grounds remains a key part of immigration machinery and, just as it did with aliens, links to arguments around social cost. Illness may:

> Represent a heavy financial burden, particularly in a country such as ours where the health and personal services are provided at public rather than private expense.
> (Yellowlees Report 1980 cited in Hayes 2000: 68)

Since the creation of the National Health Service there have been arguments about its usage by 'outsiders'. Eventually in 1982, after examples of illegal exclusion of black people from free treatment and requests for passports (Gordon 1983; Cohen and Hayes 1998), the NHS Charges to Overseas Visitors Regulations were imposed. These restrict free treatment to those deemed 'ordinarily resident' and have given momentum to increasingly sophisticated mechanisms in the NHS to ensure that free treatment is restricted to those entitled. The impact of such restrictions goes beyond the effects on casual visitors to the UK, as we shall see later in this chapter.

Social insecurity

We noted earlier how immigration restrictions were central to arrangements for social security prior to the immigration of black Commonwealth citizens in the post-war period. Since that time it has been well documented that the pattern has continued with respect to this group (Gordon and Newnham 1985; Stephenson 1989). The practice of requesting passports by Department of Social Security staff has been shown to fall heavily on black claimants, and what has emerged has been a strengthening of the link between the mechanisms of the welfare state and the internal control of immigration. Definitions of 'public funds' now include income support, housing benefit, family credit and council tax benefit, to name but a few (Shutter 1995). The 'habitual residence test' means those claimants who cannot prove the UK is their 'centre of interest' are vulnerable to the discretionary judgements of DSS staff. Research has shown, as Gordon's did in the 1980s that these judgements are exercised in a racist manner, affecting many black British citizens (TUC 1995).

Recurrent themes

Debates around the question of immigration in 1960s and 1970s Britain focused, not on refugees, but British citizens from the Commonwealth – invited guests who outstayed their welcome. British immigration policy in this period was shaped in this racist way specifically to erode the citizenship rights of this group. 'By the early 1950s the British public had warmed to a narrow definition of kith and kin' (Harding 2000: 50). Debates about control re-emerged, echoing their predecessors. Images around disease, crime and cost to the nation were replayed with exaggerated figures, running into distortions in order to create a climate of fear and panic. The culmination was the 1962 Commonwealth Immigrants Act, which marked a turning point in the status of black people who had previously had British citizenship. 'A British citizen was not completely a British citizen when he was a black British citizen' (Sivanandan 1982: 108). Legislation was to follow in quick succession, most notably, the 1968 Commonwealth Immigrants Act, the 1971 Immigration Act and the 1981 British Nationality Act, which meant by the 1980s black immigration for settlement had all but ended. Throughout this, 'recourse to public funds' remained a central tenet, used by this time to stop family reunification. Dependants of people already settled could come only if they could prove they would be maintained without accessing public funds (Bloch 1997: 115).

The return of the refugee

However, what we have witnessed in the 1990s has been the shift back to a focus on refugees, as migration for settlement is no longer a realistic option. 'The spectre of immigration has not receded in Britain; it has simply taken another form. The asylum seeker is now the luminous apparition at the foot of the bed' (Harding 2000: 51). In the real world of facing choices about leaving your home, your homeland, most or all of your family; to stare poverty, loneliness, despair and hostility in the face, the distinctions are meaningless. There was no talk about political refugees or economic migrants in the 1950s and 1960s, because we simply wanted workers. The stories of those travellers in many cases would have been no less distressing than those we shy from today.

> In other words, the definition of political refugee and economic migrant became interchangeable. So that . . . British Asians from Uganda were deemed acceptable as political refugees because they, unlike the Kenyan Asians, belonged by and large to the entrepreneurial class and could contribute to Britain's coffers. 'British', 'alien', 'political', 'economic', 'bogus', 'bona fide' – governments choose their terminology as suits their larger economic or political purpose.
>
> (*Guardian* 2000b)

A culture of suspicion has been nurtured, which talks of 'bogus' and 'abusive' asylum seekers. Eerily echoing the newspapers of a century ago, the *Dover Express* launched a vociferous campaign referring to asylum seekers as 'scum of the earth' (cited in Harding 2000: 56). This peaked in the dawn of the new millennium around responses to Gypsy asylum seekers. According to the *Sun* newspaper, apparently Britain has had enough of Gypsy beggars:

These familiar strangers are regarded monolithically; their given name is a synonym for thieves and cheats. As beggars and as Gypsies they are now also emblematic of all asylum seekers: beggars and presumed cheats at the gate of the West.

(*Guardian* 2000a)

Jock Young (1999: 112) has recently described these demonising processes in relation to current folk devils, namely, criminals, drug users and of course, asylum seekers. 'The demonisation process taken to its extreme *allows* the perpetuation of atrocities . . . it permits behaviour against others quite outside what is considered normal civilised behaviour'.

The current ideology constructs the 'economic migrant' as a purposeful, planned traveller intent on scrounging from the glorious and unrivalled British welfare state, and the 'asylum seeker' as the beggarman thief; the upshot of both is the same. Both are socially costly and should be outside of normal welfare provision, which should be restricted to 'our own'. What we have seen over the last decade in particular, has been a focus on the welfare entitlement of the asylum seeker and a concerted effort to limit it, restrict it and police it.

Current provision for asylum seekers

The 1993 Asylum and Immigration Appeals Act and the 1996 Asylum and Immigration Act were introduced after a campaign in Parliament and the press which depicted 'a besieged Britain, endangered by 'sponging', culturally alien hordes' (Schuster and Solomos 1999: 62). The category of 'economic migrant' was created specifically to problematise the majority of the applicants, who were apparently using asylum law to evade immigration control. Again these applicants are depicted as gaining access to benefits and housing at public expense.

Our duties to our citizens include the duty to protect our welfare and benefit budgets and our housing system at a time of economic stringency. . . . Those who should not be here but who have got round the system by false applications are of no benefit to our own people.

(Edward Garnier MP in Parliament 1992 cited in Schuster and Solomos 1999: 65)

The 1993 Act particularly targeted access to housing, whilst the 1996 Act restricted access to child benefit, housing and other social security benefits, leaving many asylum seekers destitute and homeless. From 1996 homeless asylum seekers lost their entitlement to local authority housing under homelessness legislation (Rahilly 1998; Minderhoud 1999: 139). The Act removed entitlement to social security benefits for those who made their applications in-country rather than at the port of entry, or for those appealing, the implication being that these cannot be genuine claims. Local authorities were then forced through the High Court to provide shelter, warmth and food to asylum seekers under the 1948 National Assistance Act. It was this which began the use of vouchers instead of cash benefits, continuing the Poor Law philosophy 'the principle of "lesser eligibility" whereby those receiving assistance need to be seen to be worse off than those who are not' (Rahilly 1998: 238). Rahilly further notes that checking immigration status has become part and parcel of investigating homelessness applications. Codes of guidance issued to staff contain worrying advice, likely to result in racist application.

> Authorities should note that there are many people from ethnic communities who have lived in the United Kingdom for many years and who have settled immigration status, but whose legal status nevertheless continues to be a person subject to immigration control.
>
> (Code of guidance cited in Rahilly 1998: 248)

The 1999 Asylum and Immigration Act continues the previous trends and in many respects standardises the worst aspects of the 1996 Act. The use of vouchers will be extended to all asylum seekers. All asylum seekers are therefore, excluded from the welfare system in place for British citizens. Bloch's research illustrates the consequences of such exclusion from social and economic participation, asylum seekers will be 'further stigmatised and labelled in the localities where they live . . . and dis-empowered and marginalized by their inability to participate in any activities which require cash currency' (Bloch 2000: 87).

And still the cries are for more. With sophisticated mechanisms in place in Benefits Agencies and Housing Offices to gate-keep resources, and an increasingly integrated system of internal immigration control, drawing in many public sector workers, no part of the welfare state can now remain untouched. Further education will need to scrutinise its applicants for immigration status, as withdrawal from benefits also means loss of entitlement to free further and higher education (Hudson 1997: 121–123). The Department of Health has a growing concern about the number of 'foreigners' being treated free on the NHS. *The*

Times claims up to a third of all patients in big cities are foreigners abusing the NHS. It is apparently:

> a question of fairness to those who pay taxes to support the NHS. Britain is not a health supermarket for the rest of the world. It is time we started standing up for our citizens and taxpayers rather than being a medical soft touch.
>
> (*Times* 2000)

Subsequent chapters of this book will look in greater detail at the current arrangements for asylum seekers. For now it is enough to note the extreme consequences of a process that has been taking place for over a century – of systematically removing access to basic welfare provision from people without British citizenship.

Conclusions

This chapter has sought to contextualise current attitudes to asylum seekers, and in particular their relationship with the welfare state, by focusing primarily on the origins of the connection between immigration status and welfare entitlement at the turn of the nineteenth century. I have attempted to trace this connection through the twentieth century to shed light on the current consensus, which places those in search of refuge outside of full entitlement to a range of welfare provision. The pervading features of this are sustained attempts to portray the outsider as undesirable and consequently undeserving of welfare, and linked to this the representation of them as socially costly. What unites these features, in a wilful determination to avoid responsibility, is the theme of nation at the very heart of the function of welfare. As skill shortages in Britain move the debate into familiar territory, differentiating between those who might be welcomed as economically useful and those who might not, there are understandably activists and refugee organisations wishing to confront the negative and inaccurate refugee stereotype. They rightly point to the qualifications, skills and motivation of refugees, but:

> They are not helped by book-keeper arguments about the high motivation of the newcomer. They need a more open defence, without proviso, which makes no appeal to the self-interest of host communities.
>
> (Harding 2000: 65)

References

Ahmad, W.I.U. (1993) *Race and Health in Contemporary Britain*, Buckingham: Open University Press.

Bloch, A. (1997) 'Ethnic inequality and social security policy', in Walker, A. and Walker, C. (eds) *Britain Divided: the growth of social exclusion in the 1980s and 1990s*, London: CPAG.

—— (2000) 'Refugee settlement in Britain: the impact of policy on participation', in *Journal of Ethnic and Migration Studies*, 26(1): 75–88.

Carby, H. (1982) 'Schooling in Babylon', in University of Birmingham Centre for Contemporary Cultural Studies, *The Empire Strikes Back: Race and Racism in 70s Britain*, London: Hutchinson.

Cohen, S. (1996) 'Anti-semitism, immigration controls and the welfare state', in D.Taylor (ed.), *Critical Social Policy: a reader*, London: Sage, pp 27–47.

Cohen, S. and Hayes, D. (1998) *They Make You Sick: essays on immigration controls and health*, Manchester: Manchester Metropolitan University, Department of ACS and Greater Manchester Immigration Aid Unit.

Foot, P. (1965) *Immigration and Race in British Politics*, Harmondsworth: Penguin.

Ford, P. and Ford, G. (1957) *A Breviate of Parliamentary Papers 1900–1916*, Oxford: Blackwell.

Gainer, B. (1972) *The Alien Invasion*, London: Heinemann.

Garrard, J. A. (1971) *The English and Immigration: a comparative study of the Jewish influx 1880–1910*, London: Oxford University Press.

Ginsburg, N. (1988/9) 'Institutional racism and local authority housing', *Critical Social Policy*, 8, 24(3): 4–19.

Gordon, P. (1983) 'Medicine, racism and immigration control', *Critical Social Policy*, 13, 7(1): 6–20.

Gordon, P. and Newnham, A. (1985) *Passport to Benefits? Racism in social security*, London: CPAG and Runnymede Trust.

Guardian (1997) 'Master race of the left', 30 August: 1–2.

—— (2000a) 'The truth about gypsy hordes', 24 March, 2.

—— (2000b) 'Casualties of globalism: today's economic migrants are also political refugees', 8 August, 13.

Hansard (1901–1905) *The Parliamentary Debates*, Authorised edn, 4th series, London: Wyman & Sons:
1901 Vol. 93.
1901 Vol. 195.
1902 Vol. 101.
1902 Vol. 102.
1903 Vol. 118.
1904 Vol. 133.
1905 Vol. 145.

Harding, J. (2000) *The Uninvited: refugees at the rich man's gate*, London: Profile.

Hayes, D. (2000) 'Outsiders within: the role of welfare in the internal control of immigration', in Batsleer, J. and Humphries, B. (eds) *Welfare, Exclusion and Political Agency*, London: Routledge, pp 63–78.

HM Inspector of Aliens (1906) *Annual Report*, Cd. 3473 lxvi.
—— (1910) *Summary of the First Five Years of the Aliens Act*.
Hudson, D. (1997) 'Excluded at home, excluded in the UK', *Adults Learning*, 8(5): 121–123.
Jacobs, S. (1985) 'Race, empire and the welfare state: council housing and racism', *Critical Social Policy*, 5, 13(1): 6–28.
Jewish Chronicle (1906a), 26 January: 2.
—— (1906b), 16 February: 10.
—— (1906v), 2 March: 9.
—— (1906d), 9 March: 11.
—— (1906e) 29 June: 17.
—— (1906f), 26 October: 7.
—— (1907a), 7 June: 7.
—— (1907b), 14 June: 22.
Miles, R. (1989) *Racism*, London: Routledge.
Minderhoud, P.E. (1999) 'Asylum seekers and access to social security: recent developments in The Netherlands, United Kingdom, Germany and Belgium' in Bloch, A. and Levy, C. (eds) *Refugees, Citizenship and Social Policy in Europe*, London: Macmillan, pp 132–148.
Rahilly, S. (1998) 'Immigration control: the provisions of the Housing Act 1996 and the Asylum and Immigration Act 1996', *Journal of Social Welfare and Family Law*, 20(3): 237–250.
Royal Commission on Alien Immigration (1903a) Vol. i. Cd. 1741.
—— (1903b) Vol. ii. Cd. 1742.
Schuster, L. and Solomos, J. (1999) 'The politics of refugee and asylum policies in Britain: historical patterns and contemporary realities', in Bloch, A and Levy, C. *Refugees, Citizenship and Social Policy in Europe*, London: Macmillan, pp 51–75.
Searle, G. (1971) *The Quest for National Efficiency*, Oxford: Blackwell.
Select Committee on Alien Immigration (1889a) *Minutes of Evidence*, Cd. 305.
—— (1889b) *The Report* Cd. 311.
Semmel, B. (1960) *Imperialism and Social Reform: English social-imperial thought, 1895–1914*, London: Allen and Unwin.
Shutter, S. (1995) *Immigration and Nationality Law Handbook*, London: JCWI.
Sivanandan, A. (1982) *A Different Hunger: writings on black resistance*, London: Pluto Press.
Stephenson, D. (1989) 'Racism, immigration and welfare benefits', *Probation Journal*, 36(4): 155–158.
Times (2000) 'NHS hit by "health tourist" tide', 9 August: 8, 17.
TUC (1995) *Race and Social Security*, London: TUC.
Williams, F. (1996) 'Racism and the discipline of social policy: a critique of welfare theory', in D. Taylor (ed.), *Critical Social Policy: a reader*, London: Sage, pp 48–76.
—— (1989) *Social Policy: a critical introduction*, Cambridge: Polity Press.
Young, J. (1999) *The Exclusive Society*, London: Sage.

4 Immigration controls and class

Shirley Joshi

Introduction

A recent report concerning the recruitment of skilled workers from the Indian subcontinent to work in Britain for a period of no longer than five years for 'third world' wages (*The Observer*, 3 December 2000), together with a speech by Immigration Minister, Barbara Roche in October 2000, in which she identified a need to recruit people from abroad to fill 'high-tech' jobs, have raised interesting questions about possible future directions of government policy and the role of migrant labour in the globalised economy. Both of these raise issues for the underclass debate, which has been a continuing theme of discussions about migration over the last half century.

Barbara Roche's proposed new direction for Britain's immigration policy, allegedly required for the twenty-first century, has already been flagged up in academic literature. The argument that labour market benefits for Britain could arise from encouraging selective immigration, has been discussed elsewhere (Findlay 1994). Three elements of such a policy were proposed: meeting staff shortages through a work permit scheme; the circulation of staff in transnational corporations; and entrepreneurial immigration which could generate jobs in Britain. The second and third of these are already managed within existing immigration regulations, and the first returns to legislation of the 1960s and 1970s which introduced work permits limiting migrants to particular jobs for a specified period of time, a system which fine-tuned immigration to the needs of capital.

The introduction of immigration controls: a Government dilemma

The introduction of controls on immigration was not achieved without some difficulty. In the dying embers of colonialism and with the memories of a world war that had been reliant to a significant extent on labour and resources from the Commonwealth and Empire still lingering in people's minds, the right of British subjects to settle in the UK was to prove a difficult principle to overturn. It was clear that, if Britain did not wish to tarnish its reputation within the international community as head of a Commonwealth and Empire, it was going to be difficult to deny colonial citizens permanent settlement and citizenship along with other rights such as family reunion. Furthermore the 1948 Nationality Act in establishing a UK and Colonies citizenship made it difficult for government to introduce legislation which would limit the rights of such citizens to enter the UK. It was clear however both from the negative reception the Labour Government of 1945–1950 gave to the arrival of the *Windrush* as well as from a flurry of activity in the setting up of Cabinet Committees by successive governments to look for ways of controlling 'coloured' colonial immigration together with the administrative measures to that end, that they were determined to seek ways of limiting immigration (Joshi and Carter 1984; Carter *et al.* 1995).

However, in doing this, successive governments faced a dilemma. They had no wish to rupture the links with kith and kin in the Old Commonwealth both because they were perceived assimilable by virtue of their colour and because 'immigration was a welcome means of augmenting our labour resources'.[1] Nevertheless, by 1962 the Conservative Government had produced what they perceived to be a strong case for the legislative control of Commonwealth immigration. This appeared to run counter in economic terms to the Ministry of Labour's assessment of a demand for labour as a continuing feature of the British economy, a view supported by the Treasury, who argued that the influx of 'coloured' immigration was beneficial in that the immigrants added more to the value of the gross national product than they consumed or remitted abroad (Spencer 1997). The 1962 Commonwealth Immigrants Act, through a voucher system, whereby those with a specific job to come to or with a skill that was in short supply could enter the UK, and a residential category of unskilled workers who could be allowed in or kept out as capital required, was introduced. Although these restrictions applied to all Commonwealth citizens, those from the Dominions were able to avoid them by using the visitors' or working holiday categories which were perceived as not relevant to New Commonwealth citizens. The 1962 Commonwealth Immigrants Act discriminated not only against New Commonwealth citizens, but also against working class migrants.

The myth of the underclass

Whatever the skill and educational background of those coming to the UK, most had to take jobs at a level considerably below their potential. Nevertheless both through individual and collective struggles they were able to resist being used as a source of cheap labour, although as both Duffield and Fevre have argued, they were used in the restructuring of the labour process in the foundry and textile industries (Fevre 1984; Duffield 1988). Despite their employment in low status occupations in manufacturing and the service sector, migrant workers were part of the working class. This challenges the view of some writers (e.g. Rex 1979) who have attempted to encapsulate the particular features of migrant labour's position in the concept of the underclass. Used initially in the USA, the theory of the underclass attempted to explain why there has been both a persistence of and a growth in inequality in the context of growing prosperity. The liberal version of this depicts the poverty experienced by African Americans as the legacy of slavery which is in turn linked to the development of a culture of poverty through which habits and morals inhibit people's ability to compete successfully for education, jobs and housing (Moynihan 1967). Although this version of the underclass theory is perceived as different from the moral explanation forwarded by the conservatives, whereby increased crime, drug addiction and rising illegitimacy are seen as accounting for the position of the very poor, they both provide the basis for the view that, whether for cultural or moral reasons, the condition of the very poor cannot be successfully addressed by welfare measures. In fact the provision of welfare is seen as exacerbating the problem and creating a culture of dependency. A further turn of the ratchet was provided by Murray's proposition concerning the alleged inherent racial differences in intellectual ability between African Americans and whites (Murray 1994). No amount of effort by those with such intellectual disadvantages, or state intervention, could overcome the resultant inequalities. The racialisation of the underclass was thus complete, as well as the case against the possibility of ameliorating the condition of the very poor.

While the underclass theory has not been applied with such vigour and enthusiasm in the UK as it has been in the USA, the linking of black immigration with problems of unemployment, criminality, drug abuse and illegitimacy in the inner city, together with welfare dependency and essentialist notions of culture, have reproduced some of the key elements of the underclass argument. The theme of a potential, ever-growing demanding and unassimilable underclass was evident in successive government discussions around black immigration in the period following the Second World War, even though evidence of such an underclass was hard to find. A survey on the black population of Stepney informed the government: 'The police reports that we have had from time to time do not indicate that the incidence of crime amongst coloured people is abnormally high but it is known that these people's background renders them specially liable to temptation in these directions'.[2]

The involvement of the police in collecting information on the black population reinforced the connection between immigration and criminality. In Sheffield the Chief Constable maintained a card index of the black population in the city[3] and government reports made frequent references to alleged gambling, brothel keeping, etc. among the immigrant population. Such views which propounded the notion of a propensity to commit crimes, became an important element in the 'SUS' laws in the 1970s and 1980s. The image was of an alien, lawless and criminal drug subculture inhabiting the inner city.

Another key element in the underclass theory was the imagery of immigrants as welfare scroungers. In the context of the post-Second World War debates about immigration, the issue of migrants' entitlement to what were regarded as limited welfare resources such as housing, social security, etc., was a theme that was taken up at government level. The Secretary of State for the Colonies argued that 'social services in the United Kingdom, particularly the rights of which any destitute person can avail himself under the National Assistance Act, must inevitably act as a considerable attraction'.[4]

Anticipating the arrival of the *Windrush* in 1948, the acting governor of Jamaica in a telegram to the Colonial Office conjured up the same spectacle of migrants liable to be a burden on the state, 'most of them have no particular skill and few will have more than a few pounds on their arrival'.[5] It was a theme echoed by Labour MPs in their petition to Prime Minister Attlee in 1948 following the arrival of the *Windrush*, demanding the introduction of legislation to control immigration: 'May we bring to your notice the fact that several hundred West Indians have arrived in this country trusting that our government will provide them with food, shelter, employment and social services and enable them to become domiciled here'.[6]

In the 1950s when successive governments fought hard to produce 'a strong case' for immigration control, the reports that Cabinet committees commissioned fuelled the imagery of migrants, in one particular case Indians and Pakistanis, as welfare scroungers: 'Newcastle, Glasgow and Nottingham comment that they are not engaged in any useful or productive work but merely live on the community and produce nothing'.[7]

As was the case with allegations of criminality, it was often predicted problems rather than evidence of existing ones that had to be used to make the case for the presence of an underclass, and in turn justify the case for immigration control. The 1961 Interdepartmental Working Party Report on the Social and Economic Problems of Immigration stated that, 'the curtailment of immigration ostensibly on employment grounds would not be easy to justify because the great majority of immigrants found and kept work "without undue difficulty"' (quoted in Spencer 1997: 116). Nevertheless this did not inhibit the Working Party from surmising on the future possibilities of a growing underclass: 'It is likely to be increasingly difficult for them to find jobs during the next few years' (quoted in Spencer 1997: 119). They are 'not being assimilated and tend to become identified with the lowest class of the population (quoted in Spencer 1997: 120). In fact many of the incoming migrants in the 1950s and 1960s had skills and professional qualifications. This was further reinforced with the arrival of East African Asians who were well qualified, spoke English fluently and would have had a positive reception had they been white.

Despite all the contra-evidence to the presence of an underclass, nearly every piece of immigration legislation from the 1960s to the present has contained provision for excluding those alleged to be likely to become a burden on the state and hence a part of the illusory underclass. Gordon and Newham produced a comprehensive list of those that governments considered possible additions to welfare dependency:

> Fiancé/fiancées: visitors: students. The wives of male students and children; wives and children of work permit holders; working holiday makers; ministers of religion and members of religious orders and missionaries admitted under the permit free category of the immigration rules; business people and self-employed persons, writers and artists, people of independent means and the wives and children of those in the last two categories.
>
> (Gordon and Newham 1985)

Although the fact that since 1971 no migrant has been permitted to enter the UK without a specific job to come to and for a specified period of time,[8] and that every category of dependant is excluded from recourse to public funds, the view of migrants as a potential unemployed welfare dependent underclass is rarely absent from the debate about migration. This has been particularly evident in the growing debate during the 1980s and 1990s about asylum seekers and refugees. The reconstruction of the morally untouchable political refugee into the disguised economic migrant (Cohen 1994) and hence the argument for limiting the asylum seekers' access to benefits through a series of measures, outlined in the 1999 Immigration and Asylum Act, which prevent the provision of benefits in a cash form, again conjures up the image of a public purse which needs to be tightly closed in the face of welfare scroungers. This together with the failure to protect refugees and asylum seekers, and to provide an environment where their skills are recognised and utilised and in which they can flourish, threatens to create in the public mind the mirage of a further addition to those in the inner city who had rioted in the 1980s. However the underclass never existed except in the imaginings of Whitehall and in the requests by local authorities for assistance in managing an urban crisis which had as its cause not the presence of migrants and their descendants but the decline and restructuring of British industry, together with years of neglect and discrimination against the inhabitants of the inner city.

What there is no doubt about is that migrant workers occupy a unique position in the class structure, but one that has been obscured by the theory of the underclass. Central to an understanding of that position is an analysis of the role that migrant labour has played and continues to play in relation to capital. A number of writers have drawn our attention to the ever-changing demand for labour arising from the capital accumulation process and the impact that this has on migration (Castles and Kosack 1973; Miles 1982; Sivanandan 1982). However as Miles points out it is important to recognise the significance of political and ideological relations in determining migratory movements (Miles 1993). The developments of a racialised division of labour in the UK are a testament to those political and ideological relations. The resistance that migrant workers showed to the racism they experienced and the role that they have played in the trade union and labour movement have helped to confirm the place of migrant workers in the working class. The role of organisations such as the Caribbean Labour Congress, and the Indian Workers' Association in organising black workers in the trade union movement in the 1950s and 1960s was significant as was migrant workers' contribution to a number of high-profile industrial disputes, e.g. Woolfe's Rubber, Grunwick, Imperial Typewriters, where they fought for the right of union recognition, an issue which was beyond that of the particular interests of black workers and raised the question of the fundamental rights of all workers (Sivanandan 1982). Through such union activity as well as the migrants' individual efforts, changes in their economic position as well as that of their children has occurred. There has been a growth in a black clerical, managerial and professional class, but as in the USA it has established its niche mainly in the public sector, including the NHS and the local authority, where there remains a glass ceiling which limits their upward mobility.

Migrant labour: the case of overseas doctors

Migrants in the UK have not only been from semi-skilled and unskilled backgrounds. Migration has also included people with professional and technical skills and, as can be seen from Barbara Roche's speech, such workers are to be encouraged in the future. However their position has been problematic. The example of migrant doctors from the New Commonwealth in the NHS offers a useful illustration of how migrants have come to occupy a position differentiated from professionals who have been trained in the UK, the EEC, the USA and the Old Commonwealth. The PLAB Examination[9] enables migrant doctors from the new Commonwealth and other 'third world' countries who pass it to take up junior hospital posts, all of which are training posts. However the ones which migrant doctors are most likely to compete for successfully tend to be in the less attractive specialisms, e.g. geriatrics and psychiatry, and are in small town locations. If promotion from such posts was fairly rapid and access to the most senior positions a possibility, the costs of a period in such posts, and locations which are recognised as having poor working conditions, would not appear to be too high a price for eventual job satisfaction and monetary reward. However the existence of a two-track training programme, one which gives a Certificate of Completion of Specialist Training and permits access to 'type-A' jobs, i.e. those that can lead ultimately to consultant status and the other, a Fixed Term Training Appointment, which while it allows doctors to complete their training, only leads to 'type-B' jobs, i.e. staff-grade jobs which are categorised as non-career-grade jobs. These exclude doctors from the more challenging, interesting and rewarding work in their specialisms as well as permanent consultant posts, and divides the profession on colour lines.[10] Migrant doctors also find themselves disadvantaged by the fact that their immigration status is constantly under review and, by virtue of the six-month contracts that many of them are on, they become an insecure mobile labour force that has no option but to fill the lowest rung of the profession if they wish to remain in the country.

Refugee doctors fare no better. The recent Home Office strategy paper outlining proposals for the integration of refugees into the UK identifies a role for the National Asylum Support Service in working with professional bodies, and comments on the NHS proposals for addressing the challenges for medically qualified refugees (Home Office 2000). While some measures such as mentoring and induction programmes and assistance in the meeting of the costs of re-qualifying examinations are positive elements of the scheme, there is a need to address a wider range of issues, such as the provision of appropriate tutoring to prepare for the PLAB Examination as well as assistance in finding jobs. A number of hospitals now charge for clinical attachments, one of the main ways that overseas/refugee doctors can access jobs in the NHS, and doctors need financial support for this as well as for general living costs while they search for work. Such assistance would run counter to the government's policy on refugees and asylum seekers.

Refugees and asylum seekers: fuelling the panic

As a result of the 1971 Immigration Act all migrant labour was put on a system not dissimilar to the one we have just described, that is one in which non-patrials could only apply for a work permit which carried neither the right of permanent residence nor the right of entry for their dependants.[11] By the 1970s changes had taken place in the demand for labour both internationally as well as in the UK. A restructuring of production processes was behind those changes, with a number of them moving away from old industrial zones (Cohen and Kennedy 2000).

However, the 1971 legislation had not been passed simply as a result of changing labour requirements, but was in part a product of a racialised discourse on immigration, which labelled new Commonwealth immigration as an unassimilable alien wedge. Despite the closing of the door to migrant labour from the new Commonwealth, the debate on immigration went unabated, partly fuelled by the New Right discourse and the failure of the Labour Party to challenge this, and partly because by the mid-1980s the debate had shifted to that of asylum seekers and refugees.

The economic changes that had brought about a relocation of some production processes were part of a wider phenomenon in some 'third world' countries of debt-led growth, particularly in those countries which had an infrastructure which encouraged foreign investment. Yet others in the face of rising oil prices were to be marginalised in this process, finding that the prices of their export commodities were falling in relation to oil and other imports. There followed in the 1980s a period of steep rises in interest rates and a resultant increase in the number of debtor countries in the 'third world'. Structural Adjustment Programmes introduced and actioned by the International Monetary

Fund and the World Bank in response to the debt and bankruptcy in many countries had far reaching consequences, including a decline in the provision of food, a growth in the power of the transnational corporations and a period of great political, social and economic instability. The rapid growth in the number of refugees and asylum seekers is one of the consequences of those conditions. The collapse of many of the communist governments has added to the flow of refugees and asylum seekers seeking relief from conditions in which human rights are frequently violated.

Such vast upheavals in the world with the dislocations that it has produced and continues to produce, have fuelled the British Governments' pressure to migrate assumption, which for so long has guided and determined successive governments' policies on immigration (see Commission for Racial Equality 1985: 90).[12] The trickle of refugees, it was surmised, was about to become a flood, confirmed by Barbara Roche's assertion in October 2000 that asylum has now become a major channel for migration. Neither the fact that most of those who had experienced the political and economic upheavals of the 1980s and 1990s had the means to migrate anywhere, except to escape into the hills or over the nearest border to try to find some relief from the conditions that they were facing, nor the underlying factors that had given rise to such economic and political upheavals, were given any attention. The fact that the vast majority of those seeking asylum have been granted refuge in countries close to those from which they are fleeing has also been conveniently ignored.

The government's perception of refugees as disguised economic migrants has led to the introduction of a series of measures in the Immigration and Asylum Act 1999 which make life difficult, unpleasant and dangerous for many refugees and asylum seekers. Furthermore it has led to an apparent contradiction. The Minister for Immigration recently identified a skill shortage that faces Britain and the need to review immigration policy in the light of this. At the same time the government, steeped in the underclass discourse of illegality, welfare dependency and the unassimilability of refugees and asylum seekers, is unwilling to use the talents and skills that refugees possess.

Nevertheless Barbara Roche has recognised that in the globalised economy the ability of capital to access the workers it needs is central to survival. Despite the technological revolutions of the past decades which many had predicted would reduce the need for labour, this has not happened. Roche's speech underlines two points: first that the state has an important role in making labour available to capital, and second that they choose to do this on their own terms and with the right to send it back when it has served its purpose. Hence the preference for recruiting labour on a temporary contract basis and the bypassing of a rich vein of skills and experience that lies with refugees and asylum seekers.

The reluctance of the government to create an environment in which refugees and asylum seekers could work and flourish rests uneasily with the new immigration policy they have proposed. The government's intention to fine-tune the flexible and market-driven aspects of the current work permit system is reminiscent of the use of alien labour in the 1940s and 1950s and bonded labour from Barbados in the 1950s.[13] The recruitment of nurses from the Caribbean at City Hospital in Birmingham and from Bombay at Wythenshawe Hospital in Manchester, are just two examples of contemporary schemes. Such workers come fully trained and qualified, a brain drain from the 'third world' to be spewed out when they have served their purpose. For those who have their wages fixed at 'third world' rates of pay they will not even enjoy the few crumbs from the rich man's table that will come in the form of remuneration to high-tech workers while their contracts last. Even then, the denizens will be returned to the place from whence they came, except perhaps for the few whose wealth puts them beyond reach of the immigration controls.

The position of contract workers however transient, has some formality and legality. Those of illegal and undocumented workers who meet the need for labour in areas such as agriculture, catering and domestic work do not even have that protection. They sell their labour in conditions over which they have no control. They earn very low wages, experience very poor conditions at work with no benefits, sick pay, pension and employment rights, no protection in respect of health and safety and no right to organise. They are beyond protection, beyond welfare, prey to harassment, violence and intimidation. Some European countries have regularised the position of their undocumented workers, e.g. Italy, potentially avoiding the grosser human rights abuses that such workers may be exposed to. Despite the British Government's recognition of the exploitation of its own undocumented workers the consideration of their legalisation has not even been put on the agenda.

While capital exploits the opportunities of the globalised economy, the role of the government identified by Barbara Roche is to manage those opportunities. The policies that they have chosen will continue to marginalise the migrants who have been so crucial to the realisation of those opportunities. Those polices have been underpinned by a discourse on the underclass as well as moral panics created about migrants, asylum seekers and refugees, and have had a huge cost to the lives involved. A recognition of the incongruence between such policies and a society which claims to respect the human rights of all people, would be a starting point for re-thinking our whole approach to immigration.

Notes

1 CAB 128/29 CM39 (55) minute 7, meeting 3 November 1955.
2 EO 1028/25, J. Nunn to E. Cass, 23 January 1950.
3 CO 1028/25 Police Report upon the Coloured Population in Sheffield, 3 October 1952, enclosed in Town Clerk (Sheffield), Joyn Heys to V. Harris, 8 October 1952.
4 CP (50) 113, 18 May 1950. Coloured People from British Colonial territories. A Memorandum by the Secretary of State for the Colonies.
5 PRO CO 876/88. Telegram from the Acting Governor in Jamaica to the Secretary of State for the Colonies, 11 May 1948, 'Jamaican workers for the United Kingdom'.
6 HO 213/244, J. Murray *et al.*, to Prime Minister, 22 June 1948.
7 CWP (53) 10. Working Party on coloured people seeking employment in the UK. Information obtained from the police about coloured communities in the UK. Note by the Home Office.
8 Spencer (1997: 143) argues that in practical terms the 1971 Act had little effect on immigration flows, as the 1962 and 1968 Acts had virtually brought an end to primary migration. However the Act was of symbolic significance, putting an end to the categories of alien and British subject, and replacing them with the racially defined categories of 'patrial' and 'non-patrial'.
9 Professional and Linguistic Assessment Board Examination which assesses foreign trained doctors' knowledge of English and medical expertise. They have to pass this to enable them to register with the General Medical Council, which is required in order to practise medicine in the UK.
10 Overseas doctors, particularly those on the Overseas Doctors Training Scheme, are generally only accepted for 'type-B' jobs, except in those specialisms where there is a shortage of applicants from doctors trained in the UK.
11 Overseas doctors are allowed to bring in dependent wives, providing that no recourse to public funds is made on their behalf.
12 The Commission for Racial Equality identified the argument that under-pinned official thinking on the administration of immigration control as pressure to migrate, i.e. that attempts to evade immigration controls will vary in accordance with the economic and other incentives people have to emigrate from their own countries and to settle in the UK. Official thinking saw this as applying only to 'third world' countries.
13 This was a scheme organised by the Department of Health to bring workers from Barbados to work as domestics in hospitals for a specified period before being required to return to Barbados. Many left their employment before their bond was redeemed, causing consternation among civil servants.

References

Carter, B., Harris, C. and Joshi, S. (1993) 'The 1951–55 Conservative Government', in W. James and C. Harris, *Inside Babylon,* London, Verso.

Castles, S. and Kosack, G. (1973) *Immigrant Workers and Class Structure in Western Europe*, London: Oxford University Press.

Cohen, R. (1994) *Frontiers of Identity*, London: Longman.

Cohen, R. and Kennedy, P. (2000) *Global Sociology,* London: Macmillan.

Commission for Racial Equality (1985) *Immigration Control Procedures: report of a formal investigation*, London: CRE.

Duffield, M. (1988) *Black Radicalism and the Politics of De-industrialisation*, London: Avebury.

Fevre, R. (1984) *Cheap Labour and Racial Discrimination*, London: Gower.

Findlay, A. (1994) 'An economic audit of contemporary immigration', in S. Spencer (ed.) *Strangers and Citizens*, London: Rivers Oram Press, pp. 159–201.

Gordon, P. and Newnham, A. (1985) *Passports to Benefits? Racism in Social Security*, London: Child Poverty Action Group and Runnymede Trust.

Home Office (2000) *Full and Equal Citizens: a strategy for the integration of refugees into the UK*, London: HMSO.

Joshi, S. and Carter, B. (1984) 'The role of Labour in the creation of a racist Britain', *Race and Class*, 25(3): 57–70.

Miles, R. (1982) *Racism and Migrant Labour,* London: Routledge.

Moynihan, D (1967) 'The Negro family: the case for national action', in L. Rainwater and W. Yancy (eds) *The Moynihan Report and the Politics of Controversy*, Cambridge, MA: MIT Press.

Murray, C. (1994) *The Emerging British Underclass*, London: Institute of Economic Affairs.

Sivanandan, A (1982) *A Different Hunger: writings on Black Resistance*, London: Pluto Press.

Spencer, I.R.G. (1997), *British Immigration Policy Since 1939*, London: Routledge.

5 Immigration and welfare reforms in the United States through the lens of mixed-status families[1]

Wendy Zimmermann and Michael Fix

Introduction

The casual observer and policy-maker might readily believe that the United States is neatly divided into two kinds of families: those composed of citizens who have strong claims to legal rights and social benefits, and those composed of non-citizens, whose claims to both are more contingent. American families, however, are far more complex: the number of families that contain a mix of both citizens and non-citizens is surprisingly large. Nearly one in ten US families with children is a mixed-status family, that is to say, a family in which one or more parents is a non-citizen and one or more children is a citizen. Further, mixed-status families are themselves complex: they may be made up of any combination of legal immigrants, undocumented immigrants, and naturalised citizens. Their composition also changes frequently, as undocumented family members legalise their status and legal immigrants naturalise. The number, complexity, and fluidity of these mixed-immigration-status families complicate the design and implementation of the already complicated arenas of immigration and immigrant policy.[2]

This chapter uses mixed-status families as a lens to explore the impacts of recent immigration and welfare policy reforms. We first document the prevalence of mixed-immigration-status families and discuss some of the immigration and citizenship policies that drive their formation. In exploring the challenges that mixed-status families pose for achieving the goals of recent welfare and illegal immigration reform laws, we explore how recent curbs on *non-citizens'* use of public benefits may have the unintended effects of 'chilling' *citizen* children's use of benefits. We note how efforts to single out immigrant children for the restoration of benefits such as food stamps may fall short of the intended objectives because most children of immigrants are already citizens who never lost their eligibility for benefits in the first place.

These benefit restorations may also fall wide of the mark because the citizen children may still suffer the effects of their parents' reduced eligibility. Both of these results are, in a sense, the by-products of mixed-status families and social policies that treat citizens and noncitizens differently.

We also examine how recent laws limiting undocumented immigrants' ability to adjust from illegal to legal status could effectively perpetuate certain mixed-status families. They do so by freezing a growing number of parents and children into differing statuses: parents as undocumented immigrants or 'outsiders' – to use Peter Schuck's (1998) phrase – children as citizens or 'insiders'. At the same time, policies that make it easier to remove or deport illegal and legal immigrants could have the impact of dividing more mixed-status families. While these policies might serve the goal of reducing illegal immigration, they do so at the expense of family unity. Finally, we note that a new policy denying legal immigrant status to aliens whose sponsors do not have incomes over 125 per cent of the Federal poverty level, could have the unintended effects of either keeping families apart or transforming what might have been a legal immigration flow into an illegal one. The result, again, could be to increase the number of mixed-status families whose members could face divided fates as the parents are locked into illegal status while their children are born as citizens. The citizen children in these families may not receive the same opportunities as other citizen children, owing to their parents' legal status.

From the outset, we should make clear that we do not believe the 'solution' to the challenges raised by mixed-status families is to transform the policies that give rise to them, most notably the strong family reunification thrust of our immigration policies and the grant of birthright citizenship. Our aim, rather, is to call attention to the unintended effects of social policies such as welfare reform, that do not appear to take into account the mixed legal statuses of immigrant families and the prevalence of citizen children within them when public benefits and rights are partitioned.

The importance of mixed-immigration-status families

Mixed families' demographic importance

A review of the 1998 Current Population Survey (CPS) reveals that mixed-status families are surprisingly prevalent. Nine per cent of US families with children are mixed-status families. Not surprisingly, such families are more prominent in the places where immigrants are concentrated. Over a quarter of California families with children, and 14 per cent of New York families with children, are mixed-status families. At the same time, 85 per cent of immigrant families (i.e. those with at least one non-citizen parent) are mixed-status families. The meaning of this is clear: *most policies that advantage or disadvantage noncitizens are likely to have broad spillover effects on the citizen children who live in the great majority of immigrant families.*

The demographic importance of mixed-status families is made even clearer by the number of children who live within them. One in ten children in the United States lives in a mixed-immigration-status family.[3] One-quarter of all children in New York City and nearly half of all children in Los Angeles live in mixed families. That such a surprisingly large share of children live in mixed families stems from the fact that non-citizens are more likely to live in families with children, and non-citizens' families contain more children. According to the 1998 Current Population Survey (CPS), 54 per cent of households headed by non-citizens have at least one child in them, versus 36 per cent for their citizen counterparts (Fix and Passel 1999). Families with at least one non-citizen parent have an average of 2.04 children, while families with only citizen parents have an average of 1.86 children. Of course, high levels of immigration in recent years have also contributed to the growing numbers of mixed-status families and to the number of children who live within them.

The significance of mixed-status families for social welfare policy

Beyond their straightforward demographic importance, mixed-status families are significant because they are more likely to be poorer than other families and hence to be of concern to social welfare policy. While mixed-status families make up 9 per cent of all families with children nationwide, they constitute 14 per cent of all such families with incomes under 200 per cent of the federal poverty level. Again, they are especially common in regions where immigrants are concentrated. Mixed-status families represent 40 per cent of low-income families with children in California and 20 per cent of such families in New York state. Nearly three-fifths of low-income children in Los Angeles and one-third of low-income children in New York City live in mixed-status families. Mixed-status families also account for a substantial share of children without health insurance: 21 per cent of all uninsured children nationwide and over one-half of California's uninsured children live in mixed families.[4]

The significance of mixed-status families in partitioning citizen versus alien rights

A third reason mixed-status families are important is because they redefine the legal and equity issues to which recent welfare and illegal immigration laws give rise. It could be argued, for example, that welfare reform has created two classes of citizen children. One class lives in households with non-citizens and suffers the disadvantage of losing benefits and the reduced overall household resources that may result; a second class of citizen children lives in households with only citizens and suffers no comparable disadvantage. The emergence of these two classes of citizen children poses the question whether their differing eligibility for benefits should be viewed as an example of constitutionally acceptable discrimination against aliens or as a more problematic instance of unacceptable discrimination between similarly situated citizens. In short, the presence of so many citizens in families with non-citizens suggests that recent reforms should be viewed through a lens of *alien rights* as well as one of *citizen rights*, which are substantially broader and more robust constitutionally (Motomura 1997).

Fundamental elements of citizenship and immigration policy drive the creation of mixed-status families

The number of mixed-status families can be ascribed in large measure to two structural elements of US citizenship and immigration policy. One is birthright citizenship. The other is immigration policy's abiding commitment to the goal of family unification and, in particular, the principle that citizens should be able to unite with immediate family members more or less as of right. A third feature of recent policy should also be noted: the proliferation of permanent and temporary immigration statuses, which creates new and more complicated types of mixed-status families. The importance of each of these factors is reinforced by high, continuing levels of legal and illegal immigration.

Birthright citizenship

The framers of the Fourteenth Amendment to the Constitution, seeking to vest the recently emancipated slaves with US citizenship, granted citizenship to 'all persons born or naturalized in the United States'.[5] The amendment confers citizenship status on all persons born on US soil, whether their parents are legally present or not. While some scholars have claimed that the framers did not intend to confer membership on the children of undocumented aliens (see Schuck and Smith 1985), their view remains a minority one.[6] Moreover, the constitutional, as opposed to legislative, basis of the doctrine makes it unlikely to be disturbed, despite repeated legislative efforts to overturn it.

The grant of birthright citizenship is a defining feature of US immigration, civil rights, and family law, aligning the United States with other nations that confer citizenship on the basis of place of birth *(jus soli)* and distinguishing it from countries where citizenship derives solely from family heritage *(jus sanguinis)*. Because most children of US immigrants are born in the United States, birthright citizenship largely explains the fact that three-quarters of children in immigrant families (i.e. families with a non-citizen parent) are citizens.[7] Eighty-nine per cent of the children in mixed-status families (i.e. families with a non-citizen parent and a citizen child) are citizens.

The birthright citizenship provision gives rise to two distinct and predominant types of mixed-status families: those with an illegal immigrant adult and a citizen child, and those containing a legal immigrant parent and a citizen child. A 1998 study of the immigrant population in New York that imputes legal status to the foreign born finds that 22 per cent of all mixed-status family households are headed by an undocumented immigrant and that one-third of all undocumented-headed households in New York contain citizen children. Of those undocumented-headed households with children, 70 per cent contain a native-born child (Passel and Clark 1998). Citizen children, then, predominate, even in families headed by an undocumented immigrant.

Mixed families containing undocumented adults and citizen children and those containing legal immigrant adults with citizen children raise distinct and common issues.[8] Both types of family may be reluctant to apply for public benefits for citizen children. Illegal immigrants are likely to fear detection and deportation, or worry that use of services by their citizen children will prevent them from eventually adjusting to legal immigration status. Legal immigrant parents may also be 'chilled' from applying for public benefits for their children, but their reasons may differ. They may be concerned that benefit use will trigger a claim for repayment on the part of government, or keep them from successfully sponsoring a relative for admission to the United States.[9] Or they may erroneously believe that benefit use on the part of their citizen children can bar them from naturalising.

Family unification

A second structural element of US immigration policy that gives rise to mixed-status families (but in a quite different way) is the goal of family unification that has dominated immigration policy at least since 1965. Of particular consequence is the hitherto unrestricted right of citizens to unite with their immediate family members (i.e. spouses, minor children, parents), which in practice, has meant that most immigrants entering the United States as legal permanent residents join citizen family members. As one scholar has written:

> The United States is committed to the principle that its citizens may both marry anyone they wish (excepting, of course, minors and persons of certain very close degrees of consanguinity) and live with that person in the United States if they so wish.[10]
>
> _   (Jasso 1996)

In fact, over half of the approximately 800 000 immigrants admitted in FY (fiscal year) 1997 came to join a US citizen family member, with the remainder entering to unite with a legal permanent resident, for employment purposes, or as a diversity immigrant.[11] The largest single category of family or any other type of immigrant admitted is spouses of US citizens. Immigrants entering under the Immigration and Naturalization Act's family unification provisions are, by and large, young and most often have US-born citizen children after arriving in the United States, creating mixed-status families. Of course, the continuing high levels of immigration to the United States ensure the ongoing creation of large numbers of mixed families.

The admission of a large number of spouses as immigrants, in turn points to another feature of mixed families: the mixed status of parents. A slightly larger share of mixed families is made up of a citizen parent and a non-citizen parent than of two non-citizen parents (41 per cent versus 39 per cent). But even when both parents are noncitizens, a large majority of their children (83 per cent) are citizens.

Proliferation of immigration statuses

A third feature of recent US immigration policy that has led to the creation of additional types of mixed-status families is a proliferation in immigration statuses assigned to entrants. These statuses, which generally fall in between the classification of legal permanent resident (or green card alien) and undocumented alien, frequently allow non-citizens to work and live in the United States, but not to naturalise. In some instances, the status is premised upon an assumption that the migrant's tenure is temporary. An example is entrants granted temporary protected status who cannot return to their home country because of political turmoil or natural disasters. (In other cases, no assumption that the stay will be only temporary is made; an example is aliens who have been paroled into the country for humanitarian reasons.) These statuses have often been the by-product of immigration emergencies that have forced ad hoc accommodations in order to admit or to avert the deportation of those with strong equities in the country. Of course, children born in the United States to immigrants in these in-between categories are citizens and, thus, generate yet a different type of mixed-status family.[12]

It goes without saying that not all citizenship and immigration policies promote the creation of mixed families. One set of policies that moves in the opposite direction is those that make naturalisation comparatively easy, at least by international standards. Several aspects of naturalisation policy should be noted. One is the comparatively short period of residence that is required: three years for the spouses of citizens, five years for others.[13] Another is the automatic conferral of citizenship status on minor children when both parents have naturalised. A third is the comparatively modest level of language and civics knowledge that is demanded of naturalisation applicants.[14] At the same time, while the goal of policy can be seen as making naturalisation accessible, administrative inefficiencies in adjudicating naturalisation benefits have led to lengthy waiting periods and delayed legal immigrants' ability to convert their status.

Mixed families and the transformation of immigration law

As we have seen, several foundational elements of immigration and citizenship policy drive the creation of mixed-status families. Beyond these structural features, the number and fates of mixed-status families have been affected by other, largely liberalising, trends in immigration law and policy that emerged in the 1970s and 1980s. These trends extended the due process norms that had been well established in other domains of US public law to immigration. In practice, they set the non-citizen and citizen members of mixed-status families on a more even footing when it comes to the claims they can make on society. But immigration law and policy evolve in an epiphenomenal manner. And just as the liberalising expansions of rights of the 1970s and 1980s represented something of a reversal of the comparatively harsh immigration policies that preceded them, they, in turn, appear to have been reversed by the largely exclusionary legislation enacted by Congress in 1996. Rather than aligning the differing fates of members of mixed-status households, the new laws deepen divisions within them.

Liberalising trends of the 1970s and 1980s

In part as a result of Supreme Court doctrine that emerged in the 1970s, it became clear that the states did not have the authority to discriminate on the basis of alienage in their public benefit programmes.[15] While the Federal government might retain this power to discriminate, there was little political impetus to do so, and until the mid-1990s few distinctions were drawn.[16] It could be argued that, by treating legal immigrants on a par with citizens, Federal policy effectively discounted the importance of citizenship. As a result, citizenship distinctions were largely restricted to voting, holding political office, serving on juries, sponsorship of immediate family members, holding some public-sector jobs, and exposure to deportation. All these are important to be sure, but they are not critical aspects of daily membership in the society. The net effect had been only modest incentives to naturalise and, by extension, a proliferation of mixed-status families. Notwithstanding this proliferation, naturalisation rates in the United States are quite high by international standards. According to the INS, almost half of immigrants admitted in 1977 had been naturalised by 1995 (US Immigration and Naturalization Service 1997).

Other policies, also in large part the product of judicial doctrine, muted distinctions based on immigration status. Perhaps the most striking and inclusionary was the grant of the substantive right to elementary and secondary education extended to undocumented children by the landmark 1982 Supreme Court decision *Plyler v. Doe*.[17] When viewed through the lens of mixed-status families, this ruling eliminated critical differences in the rights and treatment of legally present and undocumented children who happen to be members of the same family. Again, legally distinct members enjoyed comparable substantive rights.

Along similar lines, courts extended new procedural rights to aliens in the process of being deported (see for example Schuck 1998). They also mandated the extension of some public benefits to immigrants falling in the 'in-between' immigration statuses mentioned in the preceding section.[18] These and other rulings that extended new procedural and substantive rights to non-citizens effectively softened the distinctions in the treatment of immigrants in differing legal statuses. Viewed as a whole, these rulings on benefits eligibility, relief from deportation, and illegal immigrants' rights to education turned in part on the duration and depth of immigrants' ties to their communities and families. They were also driven to some degree by a new willingness to apply communitarian or universalistic principles to the cases presented by aliens (on this point and on the epiphenomenal character of immigration law generally, see Schuck's 1984 classic article). In the process, they blurred the formal legal distinctions between citizens and legal non-citizens, and to a more limited extent, between legal and illegal non-citizens.

Against this backdrop of a largely court-formulated expansion of non-citizens' rights and benefits, Congress in 1986 sought to reduce the size of the illegal immigrant population in the United States by enacting a legalization programme that eventually granted legal status to 2.8 million formerly illegal immigrants. The majority of those legalised under the law (the 1986 Immigration Reform and Control Act, or IRCA)[19] had been in the United States for at least five years, and a large share had native-born US children.[20] Soon thereafter, Congress enacted the 1990 Immigration Act, expanding legal immigration by 40 per cent and retaining family unification as a central goal of immigration policy.[21] At the same time, in what can be considered one of the few *de facto* acknowledgements of mixed-status families under immigration law, Congress granted work authorisation to, and barred the deportation of, certain undocumented family members of immigrants who had legalised under IRCA.

The exclusionary policies of 1996

A harsh California recession, unabated levels of illegal immigration, and the emergence of immigration and welfare use among immigrants as wedge issues led Congress in 1996 to enact an unprecedented tough legislative agenda that substantially restricted the legal and social rights of immigrants. As enacted, welfare reform or the Personal Responsibility and Work Opportunity Reconciliation Act of 1996 (PRWORA) transformed immigrant policy by:

• Barring most immigrants from food stamps and Supplemental Security Income (SSI), cash assistance for the poor, elderly, and disabled. Immigrants barred from these programmes included 'current' immigrants who were already in the United States at the time the law was enacted and new 'future' immigrants who had yet to enter.

- Barring new immigrants for five years from Federal means-tested benefits, defined so far to include Temporary Assistance for Needy Families (TANF), Medicaid, and the Child Health Insurance Program (CHIP).
- Giving States the option of barring current immigrants (i.e., those in the United States on or before 22 August 1996) from TANF, Medicaid, and the Social Services Block Grant. The law also gave states the option of barring new immigrants (arriving after 22 August 1996) from TANF and Medicaid following a mandatory five-year bar. In so doing, the Congress seemed to depart from prior Supreme Court rulings that barred states from discriminating against legal immigrants in determining eligibility for certain federal, state, and locally funded benefit programmes (no express grant of Congressional authority to discriminate had been in place in the earlier cases presented to the Court.)
- Exempting some legal immigrants with strong equities from the benefit restrictions. These include refugees during their first several years in the United States, legal immigrants who have worked for 10 years or whose spouse or parents have done so, and non-citizens who have served in the US military.
- Barring immigrants not considered qualified from all Federal public benefits and requiring that public agencies that dispense them verify the legal status of applicants.[22] Unqualified immigrants include not only undocumented aliens, but also other groups with authority to remain in the United States without permanent residence, some of whom had been determined to be eligible for selected federal benefits by the courts.[23]

The Antiterrorism and Effective Death Penalty Act[24] and the Illegal Immigration Reform and Immigrant Responsibility Act of 1996,[25] both passed in the same year as welfare reform, scaled back the rights of legal and illegal immigrants in far-reaching ways. They:

- Mandate the deportation of legal permanent residents and illegal immigrants for relatively minor crimes, withdrawing discretion from immigration judges to consider the resulting hardship on family members.[26]
- Limit judicial review available to immigrants facing deportation or removal or seeking waivers to the new barriers of admissibility.[27]
- Raise the 'hardship' standards non-citizens have to meet to win relief from deportation (referred to as cancellation of deportation) by extending from seven to ten years the required length of US

residence and by introducing a new annual cap of 4000 where no previous limit existed.[28]

- Introduce new expedited removal and summary exclusion measures that apply to migrants arriving without papers or with false or invalid papers and to illegal immigrants residing in the United States for less than two years.[29] Migrants who are summarily excluded have no rights of appeal and are barred from entering for five years.

- Make it harder for persons who had resided in unauthorised status to re-enter the country, barring for three years those in the United States for more than six months and for ten years those in the country more than a year.[30] These barriers to entry, in conjunction with the 'sunset' of the provision that made it possible for illegal immigrants to adjust their status without returning to their home country, effectively foreclose the ability of the undocumented to gain legal status.[31]

Some of the reforms noted above (in particular those that make it easier to deport, remove, or bar immigrants from the United States) may have the effect of dividing mixed-status families. Other provisions, which complicate or foreclose adjustment from illegal to legal to citizenship status, may have the effect of freezing mixed-status families into differing statuses: dividing the fates of family members, if not the families themselves, with potentially negative effects on citizen children.

A third major policy shift in 1996 introduces a powerful back-door reform to legal immigration policy. The illegal immigration reform law imposed for the first time a minimum income requirement on legal immigrants' sponsors that exceeds the poverty line, making it more difficult for individuals and families to bring a relative (including a spouse) to live in the United States.[32] In addition to this higher income level required of sponsors, the new law requires stronger documentation of income (i.e. the three most recent years of Federal tax returns) and forecloses taking into account the income of a spouse unless he or she has been living in the household for at least six months. The law also requires sponsors to promise to support the incoming immigrants (if they cannot support themselves) until the immigrants have worked for ten years or become citizens.[33] Sponsors are also held liable for repayment of certain benefits that may have been used during that time.

Mixed families and the implications of welfare and immigration reforms

Viewed through the lens of the mixed family, the 1996 welfare and illegal immigration reforms have far-reaching and, in some instances, unexpected implications for immigrants and their families, for the number of mixed families, and for public policy. Some effects can already be documented, but the full impact of these laws remains somewhat speculative.

Divided fates

As mentioned, the prevalence of mixed-status families means that when the law draws sharp distinctions between citizens and non-citizens it ends up treating members of the same family quite differently. Under welfare reform, for example, legal immigrants entering the United States after 22 August 1996, are barred from Medicaid for their first five years in the United States. As a result, a legal immigrant child who entered the United States two years ago would not be eligible for Medicaid, but her US-born citizen brother would be, even though both live in the same household and have the same resources available to them. The older child's lack of health insurance will mean that she has less access to preventive and other forms of health care than her sibling.

Spillover effects

While benefit restrictions may explicitly target non-citizens, they inevitably affect citizen family members as well. Take for example, current law governing non-citizens' access to food stamps. When Congress barred non-citizens from food stamps, citizen children remained eligible, but their non-citizen parents did not. Food stamps, though, are provided on a household, not an individual, basis. That is, the amount of food stamps received is based on the number of eligible people in the household. Thus, mixed-family households, along with the citizen children in them, receive fewer food stamps than they did before the cuts and presumably have less to eat.

Spillover effects can also be seen in mixed families' declining use of public assistance, despite their continued eligibility. Falling benefit use in these households occurs in large measure because of the chilling effects of shifting eligibility requirements, uncertain and sometimes over-broad application of the public charge provisions,[34] and the unfathomable complexity of the new rules regarding immigrant eligibility for benefits. The steep decline that we see in programme participation within these households is not confined to their non-citizen members, but spills over to citizen children.

Data from Los Angeles County show that approved applications by non-citizen-headed families for welfare and Medi-Cal dropped by 52 per cent between January 1996 and January 1998; there was no change for citizen families.[35] Most of the children in these immigrant families are citizens. This decline occurred despite the fact that California had not changed its eligibility rules for non-citizens (Zimmermann and Fix 1998). National data on benefit participation rates tell a similar story. Even though eligibility had changed for only a very few,[36] use of welfare (TANF, SSI, or General Assistance) by non-citizen-headed households fell by 35 per cent between 1994 and 1997, but the drop was only 14 per cent among citizen-headed households (Fix and Passel 1999). This same trend can be observed in Medicaid and food stamp use.

Since 85 per cent of non-citizen households with children contain citizen children, these declines in non-citizen household participation in benefit programmes are clearly affecting large numbers of citizen children. Further, the presence of citizen children does not seem to diminish these chilling effects. The decline in benefit participation from 1994 to 1997 for US households in which all children are non-citizens is not statistically different from the drop for families where there is at least one citizen child (Fix and Passel 1999). These findings are supported by an analysis of changes in the food stamp programme that compares the decline in participation of children living in native-born families with the decline among citizen children living in families containing legal immigrants. Use of food stamps by the latter group fell by 37 per cent from FY 1996 to September 1997, while use by the former group fell by only 15 per cent (Genser 1998).

Recent federal guidance defining the public charge provisions in immigration law should eliminate some of the confusion that has led to these declines.[37] The new rules define a public charge as a non-citizen who has become or is likely to become primarily dependent on the government for subsistence. The guidance clarifies the reach of public charge by drawing several important distinctions:

- For the most part, only immigrants applying for a green card and some non-citizens re-entering the United States after six months abroad must demonstrate they will not become a public charge. Public charge will not be taken into account when non-citizens apply to naturalise and will only rarely be grounds for deportation.
- A public charge determination will arise only from the use of such cash welfare benefits as TANF and SSI; use of non-cash benefits, such as Medicaid or food stamps will not trigger a public charge determination.[38]
- Use of welfare benefits by the family members of green card applicants will not be considered when making a public charge

determination, except in the rare circumstance where those benefits are the family's only source of support.

• Public charge will not be applied to refugees and other immigrants admitted for humanitarian reasons.

New barriers to illegal immigrants' ability to adjust status create another kind of possible spillover effect.[39] Under the new rules, undocumented immigrants are likely to remain longer in an illegal status. As a result, citizen children in these mixed families could exhibit less intergenerational mobility than they would have if their parents had been able to legalise easier or faster. While some may argue this is an acceptable trade-off to help control illegal immigration, it is a trade-off that is thrown into sharper relief by acknowledging the prevalence of citizen children in these mixed-status families. It is also a trade-off that was not publicly debated in connection with the passage of illegal immigration reform in 1996.

Public benefit restorations to immigrant children: falling short

Since 1996, the federal government has restored selected public benefits to legal immigrants.[40] The restorations go some distance toward putting citizens and non-citizens who arrived before 22 August 1996, on more equal footing.[41] However, efforts such as the food stamp restorations that targeted non-citizen children already in the United States may be, in the end, more symbolic than real because of the prevalence of mixed-status families. Three-quarters of the children in immigrant families are citizens whose eligibility for benefits did not change. Since the food stamp restorations did not cover non-citizen parents, they remain ineligible, and their households continue to receive reduced benefits. The limited reach of the restored benefits is suggested by the fact that only 29 per cent of families with a non-citizen parent have a non-citizen child, compared with the 85 per cent that have at least one citizen child.[42] Further, the impact of the restorations targeting non-citizen children will become increasingly limited over time as those children turn eighteen and 'age out' of their eligibility.

Dividing families

The new reforms depart from the historically central goal of family unification embedded in US immigration policy. Under the new illegal immigration law, all family-based immigrants must have sponsors with incomes equal to 125 per cent of the poverty level.[43] A high proportion of mixed families is not likely to meet the new income threshold: one-third of all mixed families have incomes under 125 per cent of the Federal poverty level. An even larger share (45 per cent) of mixed families where there are no citizen parents will be unable to meet the threshold.

By keeping legally present, low-income immigrants and citizens from bringing their spouses to the United States, the law may be transforming what might have been a legal immigration flow into an illegal one. The law can also be seen as further diminishing the right of low-income legal permanent residents and citizens to marry and live in the United States with whomever they choose. Thus, policies intended to increase non-citizens' self-sufficiency could have the unintended effect of abridging citizens' rights.

In a similar fashion, reforms that make it easier to deport or remove aliens in unauthorised status and aliens who have committed crimes (possibly many years earlier) are likely to divide immigrant families. Mixed families with an undocumented parent are faced with a tough choice: (i) leave the United States with the whole family, including US-born citizen children; (ii) have only the unauthorised parent leave, creating a single-parent family in the United States; or (iii) remain in the United States as an intact family, at the risk of getting caught and deported and then not being able to re-enter for three or ten years. The difficult choices faced by these families point to the inherent tension between the goals of controlling illegal immigration and the effects of birthright citizenship.

Another recent reform acknowledges that many immigrants subject to deportation have citizen family members, but emphasises enforcement goals over family unity. Prior to the 1996 law, immigrants could attempt to avoid deportation if they could prove that deportation would cause them or their family members 'extreme hardship'.[44] One factor considered was whether an immigrant had a US-born citizen child. The new law toughens the standard for what is now called cancellation of removal by requiring that immigrants prove that their removal would cause 'exceptional or extremely unusual hardship' to a citizen or permanent resident spouse, parent, or child. The framers of this new law spelled out that

> the alien must provide evidence of harm to his spouse, parent, or child substantially beyond that which ordinarily would be expected to result from the alien's deportation. . . . Similarly, showing that an alien's United States citizen child would fare less well in the alien's country of nationality than in the United States does not establish 'exceptional' or 'extremely unusual' hardship and thus would not support a grant of relief under this provision.[45]

The legislation's goal is to make it easier to deport criminal and ille-gal aliens and to ensure that an alien parent not 'derive immigration benefits through his or her child who is a United States citizen'. Again, while these may be legitimate enforcement goals, to the extent that they lead to more divided families and to citizen children being forced to leave the country they were born in, they raise questions about family policy and citizen, as well as alien, rights.

A de facto *reduction in mixed families*

Viewed collectively, the welfare and illegal reform bills may have the *de facto* effect of reducing the number of mixed families. By limiting ben-efits to legal immigrants and by exposing them to a greater threat of deportation, they create an incentive to naturalise, presumably increas-ing the number of families composed only of naturalised citizens.

Naturalisations have increased in recent years, climbing from 434 000 in 1994 to over 1 million in 1996 (US Immigration and Naturalization Service 1997). The number of immigrants naturalising exceeded the number admitted for the first time in 1996. While naturalisations are on the rise, there is still a substantial backlog of people who are waiting to become citizens. In some places, the waiting period can last up to two years, extending the time that families are in a mixed-status. In addition, naturalisation denials have increased in recent years. According to INS data, the share of citizenship applications denied increased from 7 per cent in FY 1994 to 18 per cent in FY 1996.[46] These denial rates suggest that, despite the country's comparatively easy naturalisation process, many families may be left involuntarily in mixed-status.

In addition to naturalisation backlogs, the Immigration and Naturalization Service is experiencing less well-publicised backlogs in applications for green cards. Between FY 1994 and FY 1997, the number of pending applications for adjustment of status increased more than fivefold (from 121 000 to 699 000); (US Immigration and Naturalization Service 1999). As a result, there are more illegal immi-grants in mixed families waiting longer to become legal immigrants and remaining that much further from becoming citizens.

Conclusion

As we have seen, it is extremely difficult to achieve the sometimes con-flicting objectives of the nation's immigration and immigrant integration policies: to control illegal immigration while promoting family unification, immigrant self-sufficiency, and economic and social integration. Taken together, the 1996 welfare and illegal immigration reforms restrict immigrants' access to public benefits, set new income standards, and make it easier to deport criminal and undocumented aliens. In so doing, the reforms seek to control who enters the United States as well as the conditions of residence within the United States.

Further, the mixed immigration status of immigrant families and the complex interdependencies of citizen, legal immigrant, and undocumented family members make it difficult to restrict health and other benefits for non-citizens (even legal non-citizens) without having unintended effects on citizens, particularly citizen children. One effect, then, of welfare reform and, to a lesser extent, illegal immigration reform, is to effectively treat citizen children in mixed-status families as second-class citizens. Of course, one ready solution to this problem would be to eliminate birthright citizenship. But this solution would represent a radical departure from the long-settled determination of US immigration policy that the second generation will be treated as citizens and not as the children of foreigners. Its adoption would signal a shift toward the approach taken by many European nations, which treat not just newcomers, but also their children, as outsiders, thereby perpetuating a type of hereditary disadvantage that departs from US historical tradition. Another remedy would be to put citizens and non-citizens back on equal footing, by restoring eligibility for federal benefits to legal immigrants, both those in the United States before and after 22 August 1996. Their eligibility could be conditioned by the sponsorship and public charge restrictions currently in place, restrictions that are more firmly rooted in the history of our immigration and social welfare policies.

Notes

1 Support for this chapter has been provided by the Ford, William and Flora Hewlett, and Andrew W. Mellon Foundations and by a consortium of Federal agencies that includes the Office of the Assistant Secretary for Planning and Evaluation, the Administration for Children and Families, and the Health are Financing Administration of the US Department of Health and Human Services; the Food, Nutrition and Consumer Services and the Economic Research Service of the US Department of Agriculture; and the US Immigration and Naturalization Service.

The authors would like to thank Laureen Laglagron, Scott Anderson and Alyse Frielich for their excellent research assistance; Rebecca Clark for her expert analytic advice; and Jenny Genser, Susan Martin, David Nielsen, Jeffrey S. Passel, Lisa Roney and Karen Tumlin for their thoughtful comments on earlier drafts. The opinions expressed are those of the authors and should not be attributed to the Urban Institute, its board or its administration. This chapter was initially presented at the 1999 Annual Meeting of the Population Association of America. The chapter is drawn from a paper entitled 'All under one roof: mixed status families in an era of reform', *International Migration Review* 35(2), summer 2001.

2 The data used for the analysis reported here have been corrected for over-reporting of naturalised citizen status in the current Population Survey (Passel and Clark 1998)

3 While 10 per cent of US children live in a mixed-status family, only 3.6 per cent of US children under 18 are foreign born, according to the Current Population Survey.

4 Urban Institute tabulations of March 1998 Current Population Survey (CPS).

5 The full text of the relevant clause reads: 'All persons born or naturalized in the United States and subject to the jurisdiction thereof, are citizens of the United States and of the State wherein they reside' (US Constitution, 14th Amendment).

6 A forceful counter-argument has recently been made by Law Professor Gerald Neuman (1996). Neuman claims that because there were illegal immigrants before 1875, the drafters of the 14th Amendment knowingly conferred birthright citizenship on children born in the United States to undocumented parents.

7 Not all citizen children of immigrants are born in the United States, of course. Of the 2 570 000 foreign-born children under 18 included in the Current Population Survey, 344 000 or 13 per cent were naturalised citizens.

8 It is entirely possible for some mixed-status families to include one undocumented parent, one legal immigrant parent, and citizen children. In fact, such households may be rather common, given the large number of pending applications for admission.

9 State claims for repayment may not be justified in some instances. The state of California agreed to repay funds received from hundreds of immigrants who had been ordered to pay back the value of Medi-Cal benefits they had received (Freedberg and Russell 1999).

10 As we note later, this largely unrestricted right of entry for the spouses and children of US citizens has been conditioned by a recent reform that requires for the first time that citizens who sponsor immediate family members have incomes exceeding 125 per cent of poverty.

11 The 1990 Immigration Act created a new diversity category of permanent admissions to bring in immigrants from countries that had sent comparatively few immigrants to the United States in recent years. Refugees who adjust to legal permanent resident status are also included in the 800 000 admissions.

12 Non-immigrants, including students, temporary workers, and tourists, are another group whose US-born children are citizens, creating yet another type of mixed family.

13 This period is considerably shorter than the 8–15 years a noncitizen must wait to become a citizen in Germany, for example.

14 While these can present formidable barriers for many applicants, again, they are comparatively low by the standards of most other industrialised countries (Carens 1998).

15 See generally *Graham v. Richardson*, 403 US 67 (1971)

16 See, however, *Mathews v. Diaz,* 426 US 67 (1976), upholding Congress's

authority to deny certain Medicare benefits to legal permanent residents who had lived in the United States for less than five years.

17 *Plyler v. Doe*, 457 US 202 (1982).
18 *Berger v. Heckler*, 771 F. 2d 1556 2d Cir. 1985.
19 P.L. 99–603, 100 Stat. 3359.
20 A survey of the legalised population showed that 69 per cent of those who legalised after having been in the United States for at least five years had children. Although the survey did not report on the share of those children born in the United States, at least 40 per cent had children under 5 who were likely to be US born (Comprehensive Adult Student Assessment System 1989).
21 P.L. 101–649, 104 Stat. 4978.
22 'Federal public benefits' includes any retirement, welfare, health, disability, public or assisted housing, postsecondary education, food assistance, unemployment benefit, or any similar benefits to which payment or assistance is provided to an individual, household, or family eligibility unit by an agency of the United States by appropriated funds of the United States. The Personal Responsibility and Work Opportunity Reconciliation Act, P.L. 104–193, Section 401(c).
23 The Personal Responsibility and Work Opportunity Reconciliation Act, P.L. 104–193 (1996). One objective of welfare reform was to generate budget savings. As enacted in 1996, the welfare reform law's immigrant restrictions were expected to generate 44 per cent of the law's $54 billion in expected savings, despite the fact that immigrants represented about 7 per cent of all welfare recipients (Congressional Budget Office 1996).
24 P.L. 104–132 (1996).
25 P.L. 104–208.
26 P.L. 104–208, Section 321.
27 See, for example, P.L. 104–208, Section 301, barring federal court review of the Attorney General's decision to waive newly imposed bars on admission for hardship.
28 Immigration and Naturalization Act, Section 240A(b)(1).
29 See, generally, P.L. 104–208, Sections 301–309. The measures applying to those in the US for less than two years had not been implemented as of this writing.
30 P.L. 104–208, Section 301(b). Waivers of the three and ten year bars may be granted under certain circumstances.
31 Immigration and Naturalization Act Section 245(i) permitted illegal immigrants who qualify for a permanent resident visa through family or employer sponsorship to adjust their status without leaving the country for a $1000 processing fee. In November 1997, President Clinton signed H.R. 2267, effectively sunsetting Section 245(i), while grandfathering in beneficiaries of immigrant visa petitions filed with the Attorney General before 14 January 1998.
32 P.L. 104–108, Section 551. Prior to enactment of the new law, the federal poverty level was used as a guideline, but there was no firm income requirement for sponsors.
33 An immigrant can get credit towards the ten-year work requirement from work by a spouse or parents (in the case of a minor child).
34 'Public charge' is a term used in immigration law to describe someone who

78   *Wendy Zimmermann and Michael Fix*

is, or is likely to become, dependent on public benefits. In practice, public charge considerations have historically been a factor in the admissibility of aliens (i.e. grant of a green card), but only rarely in the deportation of aliens in the United States. In the past several years, public charge has been inappropriately invoked in some instances where non-citizens have attempted to re-enter the United States and where immigrants have sought to naturalise. In some cases, non-citizens seeking to re-enter the country have been asked to repay public benefits. The legality of compelling repayment in these contexts is suspect.

35 This trend holds true for both legal and undocumented immigrant-headed families. The latter group would receive benefits only for their citizen children.

36 Many immigrants had their eligibility for SSI restored, and virtually all states kept immigrants admitted to the United States before 22 August 1996 eligible for TANF. As a result, by 1997, few immigrants had lost eligibility for these benefits.

37 See 64 Fed. Reg., Inadmissibility and Deportability on Public Charge Grounds; Field Guidance on Deportability and Inadmissibility on Public Charge Grounds; Proposed Rule and Notice, pp 28675–28693.

38 Persons in long-term institutional care that is paid for by Medicaid or other public funds may be considered a public charge.

39 These new limits on adjustment arise from the combined effects of the new barriers to reentry and the sunset of INA Section 245(i) discussed in note 31.

40 SSI and derivative Medicaid have been restored to non-citizens in the United States before the welfare law passed who were already receiving benefits or who subsequently become disabled, including some non-citizens without legal permanent resident status. Federal food stamps have also been restored to non-citizen children under 18 in the United States prior to 22 August 1996, and some elderly and disabled immigrants.

41 However, immigrants arriving *after* 22 August 1996, remain effectively barred from most federal means-tested benefit programmes until they naturalise.

42 Some State efforts to replace benefits for immigrants have employed the same targeting strategy. See, generally, Zimmermann and Tumlin (1999).

43 This new income requirement applies to most legal immigrants who enter the United States after 22 August 1996. In practice, the standard is actually even higher because the family size includes the incoming immigrant or immigrants.

44 We should note that, even before the 1996 reforms, suspension of deportation was granted on a discretionary basis.

45 Conference Report to accompany H.R. 2202, Illegal Immigration Reform and Immigrant Responsibility Act of 1996, 24 September 1996, 104th Congress, 2d session, Report 104–828, p. 213.

46 US Immigration and Naturalization Service, 1997. Another report analysing more INS data indicates that the denial rate has continued to grow and that the share of applicants denied US citizenship grew from 16 per cent in the first quarter of FY 1998 to 37 per cent in the first quarter of FY 1999 (National Association of Latino Elected Officials 1999).

References

Carens, J. H. (1998) 'Why naturalisation should be easy: a response to Noah Pickus', in N. Pickus (ed.) *Immigration and Citizenship in the 21st Century.* New York: Rowman and Littlefield.

Comprehensive Adult Student Assessment System (1989) *A Survey of Newly Legalized Persons in California,* San Francisco: CASAS.

Conference Report to accompany H. R. 2202 (1996) 104th Congress, 2d session, Report 104–828. September 24.

Fix, M. and Passel, J.S. (1999) *Trends in Noncitizens' and Citizens' Use of Public Benefits Following Welfare Reform: 1994–1997,* Washington, DC: The Urban Institute.

Fix, M. and Zimmermann, W. (1994) 'After arrival: an overview of Federal immigrant policy in the United States', in J. Passel and B. Edmonston (eds), *Immigration and Ethnicity, The Integration of America's Newest Arrivals,* Washington, DC: The Urban Institute.

Freedberg, L. and Russell, S. (1999) 'Immigrants' fears leave children without insurance: thousands have no health care in California', *San Francisco Chronicle,* 15 January.

Genser, J. (1998) *Who Is Leaving the Food Stamp Program: an analysis of caseload changes from 1994 to 1997,* Washington, DC: Office of Analysis, Nutrition, and Evaluation, The Food and Nutrition Service, US Department of Agriculture.

Jasso, G. (1996) 'Migration and the dynamics of family phenomena', in A. Booth and N. Landale (eds), *Immigration and the Family: research and policy on US Immigrants,* Mahwah, NJ: Lawrence Erlebaum Associates.

Motomura, H. (1997) 'Review essay: whose immigration law? Citizens, aliens and the Constitution', *Columbia Law Review* 97: 1567.

National Association of Latino Elected Officials (1999) 'INS makes progress on Naturalisation backlog, but denial rate increases dramatically', NALEO Press Release. March 1.

Neuman, G. (1996) *Strangers to the Constitution: immigrants, borders, and fundamental law,* Princeton: Princeton University Press.

Passel, J.S. and Clark, R. (1998) *Immigrants in New York: their legal status, incomes, and taxes.* Washington, DC: The Urban Institute.

Schuck, P. (1984) 'The transformation of immigration law', *Columbia Law Review* 84(1).

—— (1998) *Citizens, Strangers and In-Betweens: essays on immigration and citizenship.* Boulder, CO: Westview Press.

Schuck, P and Smith, R. (1985) *Citizenship without Consent,* New Haven: Yale University Press.

US Immigration and Naturalization Service (1997) *Statistical Yearbook of the Immigration and Naturalization Service, 1996,* Washington, DC: US Government Printing Office.

—— (1999) *Office of Policy and Planning, Annual Report: legal immigration, Fiscal Year 1997,* No. 1.

Zimmermann, W. and Fix, M. (1998) *Declining Immigrant Applications for Medi-Cal and Welfare Benefits in Los Angeles County,* Washington, DC: The Urban Institute.

Zimmermann, W. and Tumlin, K. (1999) *Patchwork Policies: state assistance for immigrants under welfare reform,* Washington, DC: The Urban Institute.

Part II

Immigration and welfare: the contemporary issues

6 Family life and the pursuit of immigration controls

Adele Jones

Introduction

> We all start with the presumption that the best place for a child is
> with his or her family and that the state should intervene only if
> that relationship goes wrong.
>
> (Hansard 1989)

> Family life is the foundation stone of society and we tinker with it
> at our peril.
>
> (Hansard 1989)

> . . . it is important for the law in a free society expressly to protect
> the integrity and independence of families save where there is [the]
> likelihood of significant harm to the child from within the family.
>
> (Hansard 1988)

These statements were made during the debate among politicians on the
introduction of the Children Act 1989, the primary legislation within
England and Wales governing the welfare of children.[1] They underline
the increasing importance given to family life as an aspect of social
policy. No longer regarded as a 'natural', 'prepolitical' institution
(Shanley and Narayan 1997), the family is subject to intense political
scrutiny. This preoccupation represents not so much an understanding
of the reality of family life as an expression of concern about changes
in family life, regarded by some as a collapse of traditional family life
and a cause of society's problems:

> . . . our free and reasonably successful society will be able to remain
> free and stable only when each generation moves into maturity and
> its civic responsibilities when it has effectively internalised those

values which make for freedom and stability. The only institution which can provide the time, the attention, the love and the care for doing that is not just 'the family', but a stable two-parent mutually complementary nuclear family.

(Davies 1993: 7)

The emphasis on the importance of the nuclear two-parent family promotes a narrow, orthodox view of family life and obscures the reality of the diverse and changing patterns of family life in Britain. However, it is this narrow view of family which is openly courted and supported through the existence of a range of 'penalties' for families who deviate from hegemonic ideas about what constitutes a 'good family'. 'Blaming' approaches to particular constructions of family are evident at both discursive level and in material reality and are underpinned by legislation and policy, so for example gay and lesbian parents are not considered 'good enough' parents for children in need of families through adoption, a view that has long been reflected in adoption law and which was reaffirmed during the review of the legislation (see Hansard 1993). This point is further illustrated in respect of the treatment of lone-parent families. The response to restrict access to council housing to teenage mothers, for example, on the basis that this will deter young women from becoming single parents carries a powerful sub-text – single parent families, it seems, are also not considered 'good' for children. (Ironically, within immigration practice many families are effectively reconstituted as single-parent families as a consequence of decisions made to deport or prevent entry to the UK of one or other parent.) Such views about family life are framed within arguments about morals and values which have created their own contradictions. For example, the view that the family should be a self-sufficient unit, with a shift from state care and responsibility to parental responsibility is undermined through the introduction of state regulation as to how families should behave. The principle of parental and family responsibility, a common theme which runs through all current welfare legislation seems not to be the autonomous exercise of responsibility as defined by parents, within *their* means, according to their values, abilities, resources, beliefs, etc., but a collection of duties, rights and responsibilities based on the expectations of the state. This apparent contradiction between self-sufficiency on the one hand and regulation on the other permeates legislation and policy. The Child Support Act 1992, for example, seeks simultaneously to promote autonomy in the exercise of financial responsibility for children and yet regulate where independent arrangements do not exist (NACAB 1996).

Within a study of children and immigration policy (Jones 2000), significant differences were identified between the concept of family promoted within policy and the conceptualisations and experiences of young people.

> Young people sustained connections, emotional attachments and maintained functions of care and responsibility or *did not* depending upon whether they were still *active* members of their families and where this *was* the case they were able to do so regardless of geographical boundaries. Young people's understandings suggested a *moving* between lived reality and notions of family based on remembered or imagined sets of social relations so that connections and mutual responsibilities, negotiated rather than fixed, could be sustained. The notion of the family as fluid – a set of social relations, mutual responsibility and care-giving – changing in composition and fulfilling different functions at different moments was sometimes set within traditional family forms but for other young people the social groups they regarded as family differed significantly from dominant ideas.
>
> (Jones 2000: 374)

The young people in Jones' study found that *their* family lifestyles were often regarded as invalid or subject to intense scrutiny and extensive processes of verification. Jones suggests however that, far from being exceptional to families subject to immigration controls, this conceptualisation of family may be more widely shared than that fixed on by policy makers, and that an appreciation of this by welfare professionals might lead to more creative strategies in working with children and families.

While acknowledging that the concept of the family is problematic, this chapter nevertheless seeks to examine evidence which shows that government commitment to supporting families (limited though this is), such as that given expression in the Children Act 1989, through ratification of international instruments for the achievement of the right to family life and through social policy is not extended to families subject to immigration controls. It is important here to point out that family relationships must not be the only basis on which decisions about who should be allowed entry to the UK are made, but that all such decisions should be set within a paradigm of human rights and social justice.

Within the chapter, the principal legislative and policy provisions for the support of family life are summarised. This sets the context for examining the gap between policy statements and material reality for families subject to immigration controls. Important questions are raised about whether these families are treated differentially because they have been consigned, both at the discursive and political levels to the margins of society.

Policy and legislation in support of family life

International instruments

The history of human rights developments, at both international and European level, is scattered with references on the importance of family life. The Universal Declaration of Human Rights (1948), Article 16, supports the right of people of marriageable age to marry and to found a family while the European Convention on Human Rights (1950), ratified by all members of the European Union as well as many other states outside of the EU, broadened out developments in a specific way – in that the application of the Convention should be inclusive of non-nationals who live within the territory of contracting states.[2] Although the Convention does not affect the discretionary powers of contracting states to allow a person to enter or remain in a country, where the exercise of these powers results in the enforced separation of a person from dependent children or other close relatives, such action may be in breach of Article 8 of the Convention, as has been the finding of case law (Storey 1994). The Geneva Convention on the Status of Refugees (1951) did not address the importance of family except through this reference:

> Rights previously acquired by the refugee and stemming from personal status, especially those resulting from marriage, will be respected by any contracting state, subject to the completion of formalities provided for by the legislation of the said state.
>
> (Article 12 (2))

The United Nations Plenipotentiaries Conference which adopted the Convention produced a fuller statement on the family and, while this has the status only of recommendation, it was a significant development in that it sought to extend recognition of the right to family life to refugees.

The UN Convention on the Protection of the Rights of all Migrant Workers and of Members of their Families, adopted on 18 December 1990 (as yet ratified by no member state) deals exclusively with the rights of migrant workers and draws on three texts brought together within the International Human Rights Charter and which endorse principles of family life: the Universal Declaration of Human Rights (1948); the Agreement on Civil and Political Rights (1996) and the International Covenant on Economic, Social and Cultural Rights (1996), Article 10 of which states:

> . . . the parties to this Agreement recognise that as much protection and support as possible should be given to the family, which is the natural and fundamental element of society, particularly concerning its formation and for as long as it has the responsibility to support and educate dependent children.

The rights of children to family life were underscored by the Declaration of the Rights of the Child (1959) which specified that:

> . . . to the extent that it is possible, the child should grow up under the protection and responsibility of his/her parents, and in any case in an atmosphere of affection, and of moral and material security. Young children should not be separated from their mothers, except in exceptional circumstances.

This declaration laid the ground for the UN Convention on the Rights of the Child, entered into force in 1990. The Convention addresses several interconnecting aspects of family life and highlights States Parties' responsibilities in supporting parents to fulfil parental responsibility (Articles 5, 9, 10 and 18).[3]

The relationship between international agreements and domestic legislation

With the exception of the European Convention on Human Rights, developments on the promotion of the right to family life seem to be characterised by the absence of binding powers. Furthermore, where the UK is a signatory to international agreements there may be reservations affixed to ratification which may limit the extent of compliance. This is illustrated in respect of children by the UK reservation on immigration (one of several reservations), entered on the ratification of the United Nations Convention on the Rights of the Child:

> The United Kingdom reserves the right to apply such legislation, in so far as it relates to the entry into, stay in and departure from the United Kingdom of those who do not have the right under the law

of the United Kingdom to enter and remain in the United Kingdom, and to the acquisition and possession of citizenship, as it may deem necessary from time to time.

(Children's Rights Development Unit 1994: 329)

The implications of this reservation represent a major policy factor, preventing the achievement of rights to family life as set out within international proposals since it privileges immigration controls with exemption of considerations such as the welfare of the child and also impacts upon other articles within the Convention, such as Article 3 which states that decisions must take into account the best interests of the child. As tensions and inconsistencies exist between UK and international policy, they also exist within UK policy in relation to immigration and children. These contradictions within law raise questions about the achievement of 'harmonisation' of domestic legislation with the European Convention on Human Rights, one of the principal objectives that lay behind the introduction of the Human Rights Act (1998).

Domestic legislation and policy

The Human Rights Act 1998 which is based on the European Convention on Human Rights, theoretically represents a major leap forward in addressing some of the contradictions in the achievement of social and other rights. It also makes provision for judges to consider the compatibility of new legislation with the Act, and courts will be able to declare legislation noncompatible. Although recommendations for amendments under this provision will not be legally binding on ministers, it would be politically embarrassing to pursue legislation which has the effect of undermining the Human Rights Act. The rights contained within the Human Rights Act which are relevant for the support of family life are: the right to respect for privacy and family life; the right to marry; and the right not to be discriminated against – in respect of *these* rights and freedoms. Other rights which may have a bearing in immigration cases are the right to liberty and the right to a fair trial (Clements 2000).

Children and family life

The view that children are best brought up by their families is a major principle underpinning the Children Act 1989 (Masson 1990). This is the main legislation concerning the welfare of children in England and

Wales (similar provision exists in Northern Ireland and Scotland) and it lays down the statutory duties and responsibilities of local authorities for supporting the upbringing of children by their families. Within the Children Act 1989 support to family life is given expression in a number of specific ways:

- Two important principles are advanced through Part III of the Act: the responsibility to promote and safeguard the welfare of children who are in need and to promote the upbringing of children by their families. These principles work together, so that support for children in need should enable them to live with their families (where this is consistent with the child's welfare).
- Consultation and working in partnership with families regarding children looked after and the rights of parents to be informed and participate in decisions about the child's life (Arrangements for the Placement of Children (General) Regulations 1991, Reg.3).
- The rights of parents (and children) to initiate proceedings in respect of children, that is, to apply directly to the court for leave to apply for any of the Section 8 private law orders[4] (s.10).
- The requirement for local authorities to place children who are looked after near home where possible and that siblings should be placed together (s.23(7)(b)).
- The concept of parental responsibility which a parent (who has it) does not lose, even if a child ceases to live with that parent, and if the child is looked after by the local authority.
- The principle of minimum intervention in family life, so that 'where a court is considering whether or not to make one or more orders under this Act with respect to the child, it shall not make the order unless it considers that doing so would be better for the child than making no order at all' (s.1(5), Timms 1995: 15).
- A welfare checklist in public law cases (Part IV) and contested private law cases which includes the requirement for the court to have regard to how capable each of a child's parents, and any other person in relation to whom the court considered the question to be relevant, is of meeting his or her needs (s1(3)).
- A duty to promote contact between children their parents, siblings and extended family (s.34).
- A duty to work towards reuniting children, with their families where this is consistent with the child's best interests.
- The provision of a voluntary order, the Family Assistance Order (s.16), to provide families with short-term advice and assistance where there is conflict (for example in divorce).

Although the Children Act 1989 is concerned primarily with the welfare of the child, and therefore also provides for children whose welfare may be threatened rather than strengthened as a consequence of their family life, these provisions underline the importance placed on the rights of children to family life. Furthermore, it is *this* aspect of the legislation that is strengthened by current policy initiatives which, while focusing on improving outcomes for children who may be disadvantaged as a consequence of social circumstances, regard this as best achieved through the support of family life. *Government Objectives for Social Services for Children* (Department of Health 1999) identifies key objectives for local authorities to meet regarding children in need and those in public care. Many of these objectives such as those relating to children's health, education, specific needs arising from a disability and involvement in offending behaviour are set within the context of family life. Where children do not live in families the emphasis is on ensuring that where possible they are provided with the opportunity to live within a family through increased use of adoptive placements and reducing the numbers of placement change. Significantly, the government recognises the importance of attachment and stability within childhood as factors which have a bearing on well-being and future achievement. These developments, although generally welcomed by the social work profession, raise a number of concerns, not least because they denude children of their own agency, but also because they introduce the business concepts of performance measurement and 'best value' in an area of practice that is likely to be impoverished rather than enhanced if energy and resources are consumed by the setting of targets and matching complex child care practice with performance indicators. Following *Government Objectives for Social Services for Children* and designed as a mechanism to support its implementation, the 'Framework for Assessment' introduced in 2000, requires local authorities to apply a systemic approach to the assessment of children in need[5] as the basis of the provision of family support services, with the overall objective of improving standards and consistency in practice.[6] Other policy initiatives for supporting families: the National Family and Parenting Institute; the National Parenting Helpline; an enhanced role for health visitors and Sure Start (a programme of support to children in their early years) emphasise the government's priority in supporting family life, made explicit in this statement:

> Our priority is to provide better support for parents so that parents can provide better support for their children.
>
> (Department of Health 1998)

Material reality: the impact of immigration controls on family life

Studies of immigration controls and their effects on family life (see Jones 1998) reveal major contradictions in the policy and legislative statements summarised above, and the material effects for families of the imposition of the rules under immigration legislation. What is revealed by these contradictions is that the right to family life does not exist as an absolute, non-trangressable right, and that its promotion or achievement may be subsumed where other interests are considered more important, for example, the interests that immigration controls are designed to protect.

In 1996, a National Association of Citizen's Advice Bureaux study which considered evidence from 176 Citizen's Advice Bureaux across England and Wales stated:

> . . . the extreme distress caused to the families . . . is not due solely to the narrow definition of the family in UK immigration policy. The inflexible application of the general requirements, and the highly restrictive interpretation of the 'exceptional compassionate circumstances', are equally significant elements in the overall framework of exclusion. As has already been noted in relation to spouses, the combined effect of these policies is to deprive specific members of UK society of the basic right to family life. Black and Asian families – whose members in the UK are either British citizens or have lived here for many years – are denied the rights to care for elderly relatives, or for their children.
>
> (NACAB 1996)

Defining family relationships

Discussions on the right to family life theoretically present opportunities for promoting diversity in family life. This is implied in a statement on the influence of the European Convention on the development of the concept of family life:

> Whether it is with regard to the right of residence or to the protection of foreigners who have family members in one of the contracting states from forced deportation, the study of case law clearly shows that this concept [of family] sometimes goes far beyond the framework fixed by certain national legislations.
>
> (JCWI 1993)

The statement is illustrated by examples of case law demonstrating a broader interpretation of family than may be recognised within the legislation of some member states, for example, the ruling that cohabitation is not a *sine qua non* criterion for establishing the reality of family life (*Berrehab* 21.6.88, Series A, No. 138) and the value placed on maintaining close relationships between family members, such as those between grandparents and children (*Marckx* 13.6.79, series A, No. 31; JCWI 1993).

There are several aspects of the legislation which reveal that this broader view of family is, in theory at least, supported by policy statements concerning families. In the consultation paper *Supporting Families* former Home Secretary, Jack Straw stated:

> . . . Nor is it [the *Supporting Families* consultation paper] government interfering in family life. It is not about pressuring people into one type of relationship or forcing them to stay together . . .
>
> (Department of Health 1998)

However the concept of diversity in family life has not found its way into UK immigration law. For example, the law does not include non-married couples within the definition of family; it does not acknowledge same-sex relationships; where children are able to inherit the nationality of parents, it does not allow the transfer of nationality from fathers who were not married to the mother of a child at the time of a child's birth; additional restrictions are placed on adopted children; and, there are very restrictive rules for all except dependent children and dependent parents who are over 65. (Dependent children – except children who are British citizens or others who have the right of abode in the UK – and parents over 65, do not have automatic right of abode and must also fit the immigration rules. Also, parents under 65 are not normally allowed in, even under the rules.) It is a very limited view of family which is established and reinforced. This happens at different levels and in regard to defining family relationships it is apparent that the legislative framework serves two functions: it operates both as an immigration control and also as a social control in that it promotes a particular concept of family underpinned by an ideology which is orthodox, patriarchal and based on a Western perspective. This is illustrated for example, in that while Muslim marriages may be accepted by immigration officials, Muslim divorces are often not, so that second wives and the children of second marriages may be denied the right to family life in the UK, even where they have satisfied all other requirements (Jones 1998).

Questions of recognition

The literature on immigration draws attention to particular difficulties in achieving Home Office recognition of the significance of relationships for families in which arrangements for care of dependent members have broken down and where it becomes necessary for another parent or other relative to assume responsibility. Children in this situation are subject to the 'sole responsibility' rule through which a child may only be permitted to join a parent in the UK if that parent is able to prove that they have had sole responsibility for the child's upbringing. The history of this rule illustrates the social control function of immigration rules referred to above:

> The sole responsibility rule was first promulgated in 1969. The government's stated intention was to prevent the growth of all-male Pakistani families, where men who had come to work in the UK were sending for their sons, but not their wives and daughters, and it was felt that this was not in the best interests of the children.
>
> (JCWI 1997: 51)

For a parent in the UK to resume the care and responsibility for a child previously cared for by another parent living abroad, the immigration authorities must be satisfied that either:

• The parent settled in the UK or on the same occasion admitted for settlement has had the sole responsibility for the child's upbringing;

or

• The parent or a relative other than a parent is settled or accepted for settlement in the UK and there are serious and compelling family or other considerations in the child's own country which makes the child's exclusion undesirable – for example, where the other parent is physically or mentally incapable of looking after the child – and suitable arrangements have been made for the child's care.

> (JCWI 1997: 50)

The first of these requirements is discrepant with the Children Act 1989 which promotes the concept of parental responsibility as containing the duties, responsibilities, obligations and rights in respect of a child. Parents (who were married at the time of the child's birth, and all mothers) possess parental responsibility as of right, they are not usually required to prove their parental responsibility and they cannot lose it, regardless of the exercise of responsibility, except where children are adopted. It also cannot ever be completely true that a parent who is living in the UK will have had sole responsibility for a child living abroad. The second of these requirements is for evidence of failure to fulfil parental responsibility, and this presents considerable problems since children and parents must effectively admit to neglect or abandonment:

> British high commissions also asked the children many questions about contact with their fathers, who may well have remained abroad but separated from partners and children. It was clearly hard for children . . . to admit that they had been abandoned – but if the father's contact had been kept up, even sporadically or at a very low level, this could be a reason for refusing entry clearance for the child.
>
> (JCWI 1997: 51).

The requirement to prove the validity of family relationships can be a source of distress and difficulty for some families (Guild 1994; Jones 1998). Guild (1994) discusses this in relation to the practice of DNA tests. These tests were introduced by the Home Office to provide a high standard of proof of biological relationship of children and parents where other evidence may be difficult to obtain. Guild argues that the suggestion that children may not in fact be related to their parents is one that may cause anguish and distress and, for those small numbers of families in which this is found to be the case, may create irreconcilable family problems. In 1992, of the 1043 tests that were carried out in Bangladesh, seven per cent showed the child to be related to only one parent and in 10 per cent the child was related to neither parent:

> The implications of such an intrusive measure can hardly be overestimated. The consequences for the families in those cases which revealed the lack of relationship may have been catastrophic. This is particularly the case when the child was related to the mother but not the sponsoring father. An allegation striking at the very dignity and integrity of the family can only be justified if there is strong evidence of abuse. It is not the role of immigration policy to police the fidelity of wives.
>
> (Guild 1994: 238)

However, DNA fingerprinting has also proved the validity of relationships where this may have previously been in doubt:

> During the 1970's and 80's, many thousands of children were wrongly refused entry on the basis of decisions that they were not related to the sponsor parent. The introduction of commercial DNA tests proved that this decision was wrong in 90% of cases, although by then those same children were too old for admission.
>
> (Webber 1994: 18)

Separation and family reunification

In some cases, the right of British-born children to live in the UK may lead to their families being allowed to remain with them. This was the finding in the case of *Fadele* concerning three children who were able to prove that their effective deportation to Nigeria to live with their father, who had not been permitted to remain with them in the UK following the death of their mother, had caused them great hardship. The European Commission of Human Rights ruled that the father had been wrongfully removed from the UK and the Home Office had to pay for the family's return (JCWI 1995). However cases such as *Berrehab* and *Marckx*, referred to above, which establish a principle a priori on the maintenance of family ties, do not necessarily lead to the right of abode within a certain country – on the contrary, the courts have already determined that family unity is not dependent on families living in the same household, or even the same country (JCWI 1995).

Children clearly experience hardship as the result of separation from one parent or other – this is acknowledged in the policy initiatives described above. There is evidence however, that in many immigration cases the Home Office both disregards the effects of separation on children, and of particular concern, may sometimes actively seek it.

In some cases of separation, it is the family itself who arrange the upbringing of children by extended family members separated from the parent or parents – often as a means of ensuring the survival of the entire family or of providing the best way of meeting the needs of individual children. This occurs in families where parents are unable to care for children because of poverty, work or ill-health or as a consequence of a child being sent by the family to the UK in order to escape war, as is often the case for young unaccompanied asylum seekers. These families have not disowned their children, and on the contrary often develop the means to maintain and sustain attachments and fulfil parental responsibilities despite geographical distance. It is also the case however, that some parents do lose contact with children and the children may *in effect* be abandoned.

In other cases children are separated from parents as a result of Home Office action such as deportation or detention. Jones (1998) provides examples of such cases. The first concerns two children (who were British citizens) living with a parent against whom a deportation order had been issued. In this case, the local authority was approached to find out whether appropriate care and accommodation could be provided to the children in the event of their parent being deported. In another example, the mother's chronic illness and periods of hospitalisation led to her children being accommodated in a children's home by the local authority on several occasions. The Home Office refused the children's father leave to enter the UK to care for the children or even to visit them, despite the ruling of an adjudicator that the emotional costs to the children of being placed in public care should be taken into account. A third case in which the disruption of family life was brought about as a direct consequence of Home Office actions concerned a father of five children who was deported after settling in the UK some 30 years previously. He was deported in 1995, followed two months later by the deportation of his teenage son. The effects on the family are summarised in this extract:

> When my dad was deported my life fell apart. I loved my father very much, I was his littlest child. it tore my mum apart as well, I saw her cry herself to sleep every night which made me more depressed. To make our problems worse a couple of months after my dad's deportation my brother was deported as well . . . and my brother had never been away from my family before which made me think how he would cope by himself. They even sent him somewhere different, he's in another country all by himself. I never saw them again.
>
> (quoted in Jones 1998: 13)

Regardless of the reasons for separation, key literature on child development (Howe 1995; Belsky and Cassidy 1994; Bowlby 1980) highlights the impact of separation and loss on children and young people, and the implications for welfare agencies. While there has been insufficient attention paid to the effects on children who experience separation and loss as a consequence of immigration decisions, and although theoretical positions on attachment issues are often based on ethnocentric, universalist assumptions, there can be little doubt that the impact is damaging to children's welfare. Jones (1998) found that children so separated from parents were often depressed, experienced self-blame, insecurity and extreme distress.

While there is no requirement in immigration law to take into account the effects of the separation of children from parents, this has been the subject of rulings under the European Court of Human Rights, and in 1993 the Home Office gave instructions to staff which contradicted its own immigration rules requiring them to 'take into account the effect of the European Convention on Human Rights' in immigration decisions. The instructions drew on a number of court cases which demonstrated that, regardless of the merits of an applicant's immigration history, the court would be likely to find a breach of Article 8 (of the Convention) where the effect of an immigration decision was to separate an applicant from his or her spouse or child (JCWI 1995).

Contact between parents and children

'Contact' is a term used to describe arrangements for sustaining family relationships and connections in cases in which children have become separated from one or both parents and/or siblings and extended family members. Until the advent of the Children Act 1989 which introduced a broader concept of contact, the term 'access' was more widely used and, in a legal context, this usually referred to arrangements for a child living with one parent to visit or be visited by the other in cases of separation and divorce. Contact between children and parents is also addressed through Articles 9 and 10 of the UN Convention on the Rights of the Child.[7] Most contact arrangements are decided by families without involvement from outside agencies, but in immigration cases contact between children and families must be within the immigration rules. However the application of the rules may be incompatible with the sustaining of family relationships. If a parent is deported, but wishes to remain in contact with the child through visits to the UK, for example, this is extremely difficult. The Home Office will not normally revoke a deportation order until the person has been out of the UK for at least three years, and the person will nevertheless still have to satisfy the requirements of the immigration rules to return to the UK. As a visitor, this means showing that they intend to leave at the end of a specified length of time of visit, however it may be assumed that the child would be an incentive to the parent to overstay and they may therefore be refused entry (NACAB 1996). Since October 1994, immigration rules have taken account of the rights of parents to maintain contact with their children. Persons who wish to exercise rights of access to a child in the UK must:

- be divorced or legally separated from the child's other parent
- show that they do not intend to work or do business in the UK and that they can maintain themselves without reliance on public funds
- have a court order granting them contact to the child
- show that they are coming to the UK for that purpose
- show that they intend to leave the UK at the end of the period
- have entry clearance for the purpose of contact.

While these arrangements may seek to ensure compliance with Article 8 of the European Convention on Human Rights, in reality this may not be achieved, largely because of the restrictions placed upon families through the requirements that couples must have been married and they must have court documents granting contact (JCWI 1997: 47).

Material reality: the welfare of children

The welfare needs of children, such as housing, food, clothing and education in families subject to immigration rules are, as for other children, most often provided for in the context of family life. However, several studies have shown that the ability of families to meet the needs of their children is often impeded as a consequence of the material conditions created by immigration rules. It is largely in compliance with the 'reliance on public funds'[8] rule (Immigration Act 1971) that families may be reduced to conditions of financial hardship, in some cases with damaging effects on children. However this rule is a crude and unjust measure for exercising immigration control, which results in the creation of family poverty (contravening the government's own position on the eradication of child poverty) often with severe consequences for children. Some children affected by this rule have been shown to suffer increased levels of malnutrition and other health problems as a consequence of chronic deprivation (Jones 1998). It can also lead to greater financial costs to the state in the long term. This occurs in several circumstances: where families are materially reconstituted as single-parent families (because a second parent is prevented from entering the country); where local authorities are looking after children whose parents have been deported for being in breach of this rule; where local authority provision for a child in need (under the Children Act 1989)[9] becomes necessary as a consequence of the deprivation created by the application of the public funds rule and in cases of asylum seekers who are detained for being in breach of the rule.

The general requirement within the immigration rules regarding reliance on public funds seems at one level to be a device for controlling immigration and at another appears to reflect an underlying ideology that immigrants are a financial burden on the state. Studies have revealed such perceptions to be largely based on myth and stereotype, and have demonstrated the financial benefits of a positive approach to immigration (see Runnymede Bulletin 1994; Spencer 1994).

In common with many families, families involved in immigration proceedings may need access to supplementary funds at some time or other in order to support them during periods of sickness and unemployment. It is the case however, that allowed to work and supported by benefits in times of need, families are likely to make an overall financial contribution to the state that outweighs any demand. Families, by and large, seek the betterment of themselves and their children, and they do not see this as being achieved through reliance on public funds. Furthermore, people affected by immigration controls often have skilled or professional backgrounds, with qualifications and skills that they wish to make use of. This is supported by a Home Office (1995) research study which reported that a high percentage of people granted refugee status were highly educated and qualified and many had come from professional backgrounds. Furthermore, there is the economic and skill-enhancing potential of refugees and immigrants:

> some refugees may in fact be economically highly desirable, because of their entrepreneurial potential for the host community.
>
> (Findlay 1994: 185)

While the argument is not made that immigration and the granting of asylum should be based solely on the economic benefits for British society, this is an important point since it raises questions about how and why people subject to immigration controls have come to be viewed within popular perception, as simply a financial burden on the state, and why studies which reveal this to be untrue are marginalised within immigration discourses.

Conclusion

The commitment to promote the concept of 'the family' is a major feature of UK social policy. However, this chapter highlights the absence of concern both in regard to particular types of family, that is, those families that do not adhere to traditional, orthodox family forms and also, in particular types of circumstance, even where families do conform to this notion of family life. The failure to apply policy initiatives concerned with the support of family life to families affected by immigration controls may lead to:

- disruption of family life
- prevention of the upbringing of children in families
- forcible separation of children from parents, with damaging effects on children.

These findings are clearly at odds with the government position on family life that has been discussed. Furthermore, failure to consider the impact on children of the implementation of the 'reliance on public funds' rule raises questions about the morality of policy and legislation which is designed to create privation and hardship, and which takes little or no account of the impact on children.

While there is a growing acknowledgement of the family as multi-form in composition and lifestyle, in relation to families involved in immigration proceedings, more aggressive policies seem to be at play. These include elements of political manipulation to limit claims for recognition for different family forms while at the same time promoting a unitary notion of family which is traditional, determinedly heterosexual, patriarchal and based on Western perspectives of family life. What we seem to have ended up with is a rhetoric within 'political speak' which supports diversity in family life, and practice, legislation and policy which does not. Under immigration investigations families may find that their family lifestyles are regarded as invalid or subject to intense scrutiny and extensive processes of verification. The value of family life is not solely determined by whether children live their daily lives within the family household or whether they are dependent upon families for their daily needs, yet this is the criterion upon which decisions by immigration officers are often made. There are other examples of practice however, in which parents have been deported or are facing deportation despite the fact that children, including very young children, may be totally dependent on that parent for their care and upbringing (Jones 1998).

Family life is affected by immigration proceedings in several significant ways: the separation of children from parents has emotional, psychological and material consequences; roles and relationships in some families become altered; care and protection of children, identified as important functions of the family, may be interfered with or prevented; and the imposition of conditions within the immigration rules can result in a deterioration in the material circumstances of family life. In this extract from the report of a study of the implications for children's welfare of immigration controls, Jones makes a number of policy recommendations:

. . . decisions that may result in the disruption of family life or interfere with the family's ability to fulfil responsibility for children [should only be] taken in the light of full and proper consideration of the implications for children . . . [C]hildren should have the right, *regardless* of other concerns, to have their views and the possible effects on them of separation taken into account. . . . Immigration legislation should not prevent children from maintaining contact with both parents where this is in the child's interests. . . . The general requirement within the Immigration Rules regarding reliance on public funds should be reviewed. . . . There is a need for social services departments and voluntary agencies working with children and young people to take a greater interest in immigration cases in which children are involved and where there are clear welfare implications. . . . There is [also] a need to amend immigration legislation to ensure that the local authorities' duty to promote and safeguard the welfare of children is not interfered with. . . . There is a need for regulations and guidance to be drawn up regarding local authorities' use of the provisions of Part III of the Children Act 1989 to support children in need where need arises out of immigration proceedings.

(Jones 1998: 141–143)

The absence of oppositional agency

Social work literature, policy and practice indicate an absence of critical scrutiny on the status and relationship of immigration and child care law and the contradictions highlighted within this chapter in the support of family life. There has been little attempt to challenge or deconstruct the assumptions, political aims, or policy contradictions tacit in the privileging of the status of immigration law and this may provide one explanation for the continuation of inequality, contradictions and discrepancies in the practice of immigration and child care law. Bodies with responsibility, expertise and knowledge in child welfare and child development do not appear to have considered the effects of immigration controls on children except, in some instances, in relation to young refugees and asylum seekers (Social Services Inspectorate and Surrey County Council 1995). In their failure to provide oppositional agency at discursive and ideological levels, social services departments, voluntary organisations and government bodies responsible for children's welfare, may be complicit in the creation of disadvantage and discrimination for families involved in immigration proceedings.

Notes

1 The Children Act 1989 does not apply to Scotland or Northern Ireland where separate legislation exists, however the broad principles of child care law are similar across all three administrations and it is therefore appropriate to discuss contradictions in immigration and child care law as a UK problem.

2 The European Convention on Human Rights states:

Everyone has the right to respect for his private and family life, his home and his correspondence.

There shall be no interference by a public authority with the exercise of this right except such as is in accordance with the law and is necessary in a democratic society in the interests of national security, public safety or the economic well-being of the country, for the prevention of disorder or crime, for the protection of health or morals, or for the protection of the rights and freedoms of others. (Article 8)

3 Article 5 identifies the duty of the state to respect the rights and responsibilities of parents and the wider family in providing guidance appropriate to the child's abilities and development. Article 9 concerns the right of the child to live with his/her parents where this is compatible with the child's best interests; the right to maintain contact with parents if separated from them, and the duties of the state when separation results from the actions of the state. Article 10 promotes the importance of family reunification through the right of parents and children to leave any country and enter their own for these purposes and, Article 18 rests on the principle that both parents have joint and primary responsibility for the upbringing of their children and requires States Parties to provide 'appropriate assistance' to support them in this task (UN Convention on the Rights of the Child 1990).

4 Section 8 orders are flexible orders which should be able to cater for any question which may arise about the welfare of a child in private proceedings. Replacing custody and access orders, there are four section 8 orders:

• contact order – determining whom a child should be allowed to have contact with

• prohibited steps order – an order that no step of a kind specified in the order shall be taken in respect of a child without the permission of the court

• residence order – an order settling the arrangements to be made as to the person with whom the child is to live

• a specific issue order – an order giving directions for the purpose of determining a specific question in connection with any aspect of parental responsibility for a child.

5 'Child in need' as defined within the Children Act 1989 determines the scope of local authority duties to provide services. A child shall be taken to be in need if:

a) he is unlikely to achieve or maintain, or to have the opportunity of achieving or maintaining, a reasonable standard of health or development without the provision for him of services by a local authority under this Part;

b) his health or development is likely to be significantly impaired, or further impaired, without the provision for him of such services; or

c) he is disabled (s.17(10))

... in this Part 'development' means physical, intellectual, emotional, social or behavioural development and 'health' means physical or mental health (s.17(11)).

It is important to point out here that Section 17 of the Children Act 1989 has been curtailed by the 1999 Immigration and Asylum Act.

6 The 'Framework for the Assessment of Children in Need and their Families (Department of Health 2000b) seeks to utilise best practice, research findings and child development theory within the process of assessment. There are however, a number of limitations to the approach adopted. The first concerns the theoretical base of social work which assumes that practice led by assessment of need as a means to providing services is natural, just and normative. The failure to deconstruct the process of assessment however, leaves intact the powerbase of social work, undermines the expertise and knowledge possessed by those being assessed, stifles debate on developments of other approaches to social work practice (e.g. rights-based approaches) and contradicts the principles of empowerment and partnership which are much paraded as a keystone of the framework. The second concern is that the framework contains ideas on what 'good families do' which are riddled with ethnocentric and class-based assumptions (see, for example, Department of Health 2000a). The third concern is the increase in paperwork required at a time when social workers are bemoaning the general increase in bureaucracy, and the profession is experiencing a national shortage of social workers.

7 UN Convention on the Rights of the Child, Article 9 states that: children have a right 'not to be separated from [their] parents against their will, except when competent authorities ... determine ... that such separation is necessary for the best interests of the child'. They also have the right, if separated from one or both parents, 'to maintain personal relations and direct contact with both parents on a regular basis, except if it is contrary to the child's best interests'. Enforced separation imposed by the deportation or removal of parents constitutes a clear breach of this principle (Children's Rights Development Unit 1994: 250).

8 Public funds for immigration purposes are:
   • housing under Part II or III of the Housing Act 1985, Part I or II of the Housing (Scotland) Act 1987 or Part II of the Housing (Northern Ireland) Order 1981 or Part II of the Housing (Northern Ireland) Order 1988
   • attendance allowance, severe disablement allowance, invalid care allowance and disability living allowance under Part III, income support, family credit, council tax benefit, disability working allowance and housing benefit under Part VII and child benefit under Part IX of the Social Security Contributions and Benefits Act 1992, and the equivalent Act in Northern Ireland
   • income-based jobseeker's allowance under the Jobseekers Act 1995 (JCWI 1997: 195).

9 Although there is considerable evidence that poor health and poor educational attainment are linked to poverty (National Children's Bureau 1990), the Children Act 1989 does not directly address the issue of poverty, and even where need is identified there is no duty to deal with any underlying causes. The duties identified in Schedule 2, Part I of the Act are qualified in

that the requirement to provide services to children in need is thus phrased: 'the local authority shall take reasonable steps or make such provision as they consider appropriate'. On a policy level however, many local authorities are aware that little real change can be effected to the lives of children in need unless there is sustained political commitment to addressing structural disadvantage.

References

Belsky, J. and Cassidy, J. (1994) 'Attachment: theory and practice' in M. Rutter and D. Hay (eds) *Development Through Life: a handbook for clinicians*, Oxford: Blackwell Science, pp 373–401.
Bowlby, J. (1980) *Attachment and Loss, Volume III: Loss, Sadness and Depression*, London: Hogarth Press.
Children Act (1989) London: Department of Health.
Children's Rights Development Unit (1994) *UK Agenda for Children*, London: CRDU.
Clements, L. (2000) 'Child care and general social services', *Legal Action Group conference papers – The Human Rights Act 1998 – the big picture* (unpublished).
Davies, J. (1993) 'The family – RIP? Religion, marriage, the market and the state in western societies' in J. Davies (ed.) *The Family: is it just another lifestyle choice?* London: Institute of Economic Affairs Health and Welfare Unit.
Department of Health (1998) *Supporting Families: consultation paper*, London: DoH.
——(1999) *Government Objectives for Social Services for Children*, London: DoH.
——(2000a) *The Family Assessment Pack of Questionnaires and Scales*, London: DoH.
——(2000b) *Framework for the Assessment of Children in Need and their Families*, London: DoH.
Findlay, A. (1994) 'An economic audit of contemporary immigration' in S. Spencer (ed.) *Strangers and Citizens: a positive approach to migrants and refugees*, London: IPPR and Rivers Oram, pp 159–201.
Guild, E. (1994) 'Future immigration policy' in S. Spencer (ed.) *Strangers and Citizens: a positive approach to migrants and refugees*, London: IPPR and Rivers Oram, pp 232–263.
Hansard (1988) House of Lords, Children Act Second Reading, 6 December.
——(1989) House of Commons, Standing Committee B, 25 May.
——(1993) 'The debate on the adoption law review', *Parliamentary Debates*, 3 November Vol. 231, No. 238, p 348.
Home Office (1995) *The Settlement of Refugees in Britain*, Research Study No. 141, London: HMSO.
Home Office Circular (1993a) *Instructions on Cases involving Marriage and Children*.
——(1993b) *Detention of Unaccompanied Asylum-seeking Children*.
Home Office Research Study (1991–92) CP.3.

House of Commons (Paper) 395.

Howe, D. (1995) *Attachment Theory for Social Work Practice*, Basingstoke: Macmillan.

Human Rights Act (1998) London: The Stationery Office.

Immigration Act (1971) House of Commons Paper, 395.

—— (1993) unpublished conference report on international instruments in the support of family life.

—— (1995) *Immigration and Nationality Law Handbook, 1995*, London: Joint Council for the Welfare of Immigrants.

—— (1997) *Immigration, Nationality and Refugee Law Handbook, 1997*, London: Joint Council for the Welfare of Immigrants.

Jones, A. (1998) *The Child Welfare Implications of UK Immigration Policy*, Manchester: Manchester Metropolitan University.

—— (2000) *UK Immigration Policy and Practice: a Study of the Experiences of Children and Young People*, Ph.D. Thesis, Manchester: Manchester Metropolitan University

Macdonald, I.A. (1991) *Immigration Law and Practice in the United Kingdom*, (3rd edn), London: Sweet & Maxwell.

Masson, J. (1990) *The Children Act 1989, text and commentary*, London: Sweet & Maxwell.

NACAB (1996) *The Right to Family Life*, London: National Association of Citizens Advice Bureaux.

National Children's Bureau (1990) *Child Poverty and Deprivation in the UK*, London: NCB.

Runnymede Bulletin (1994) No. 276, June, London.

Shanley, M.L. and Narayan, U. (eds) (1997) *Reconstructing Political Theory: feminist perspectives*, Cambridge: Polity Press.

Social Services Inspectorate and Surrey County Council (1995) *Unaccompanied Asylum-Seeking Children: a training pack*, London: Department of Health

Spencer, S (ed) (1994) *Strangers and Citizens: a positive approach to migrants and refugees*, London: IPPR and Rivers Oram.

Storey, H. (1994) 'International Law and Human Rights Obligations' in S. Spencer (ed.) *Strangers and Citizens: a positive approach to migrants and refugees*, London: IPPR and Rivers Oram, pp 111–136.

Timms, J.E. (1995) *Children's Representation: a practitioner's guide*, London: Sweet & Maxwell.

Webber, F. (1994) 'Home Office discretion outside the immigration rules', *Legal Action*, pp 18–20.

7   From a shambles to a new apartheid

Local authorities, dispersal and the struggle to defend asylum seekers

Ed Mynott

From the early 1990s onwards, local authorities in the United Kingdom have been affected by successive attempts by government to make immigration controls more severe. One way in which this has happened is by limiting the access of 'persons subject to immigration control' to those services and benefits (such as housing and housing benefit) which are administered by local authorities. Equally, and perhaps more importantly, local authorities have been required to provide specific, second-class forms of support to asylum seekers who have been barred from receiving the services and benefits previously available to all within a welfare state. This process began in earnest with the 1993 Asylum and Immigration Appeals Act and became entrenched with the 1996 Asylum and Immigration Act, both passed by John Major's Conservative Government. Far from ending after the election of a Labour Government in 1997, the process was intensified by the 1999 Immigration and Asylum Act.

This chapter will trace the impact of this policy of deliberate exclusion and second-class support on local authorities. It will also attempt to identify some of the key issues for those organising resistance to the forced dispersal which forms one element in the intensification of internal immigration controls.

Internal immigration controls

The history of immigration control since the 1960s is a history of increasing entry restrictions, which have been aimed primarily at black people. However, modern immigration controls have also steadily increased *internal* controls. The screw really began to be turned by the Asylum and Immigration Appeals Act. The Act introduced many punitive measures including purpose built detention centres used to lock up asylum seekers without trial or charge. In 1993 the number of asylum seekers detained inside the UK more than doubled to over 10 000 (Brown 1995: 26).

It was under the 1993 Act, that the first changes came into being which directly affected local authorities. A stricter test for assessing whether homeless asylum seekers were eligible for social housing was introduced. This was followed in 1994 by the introduction of the 'habitual residence test'. Ostensibly directed at non-British citizens (mainly from other European Community countries) coming to the UK specifically to claim certain benefits, the test in fact tended to hit black claimants, many of whom were British citizens (TUC 1995; NACAB 1996; see also Chapter 10 of this volume). The test affected local authorities because it applied to benefits administered by them, such as housing benefit and council tax benefit as well as benefits administered by the government's Department of Social Security.

By the autumn of 1995 there was a whole package of measures and proposed legislation. They were a new Asylum Bill, sections of the new Housing Bill, the Social Security (Persons from Abroad) Regulations and a study of inter-agency co-operation on illegal immigration (the 'efficiency scrutiny'; see Chapter 8 of this volume). They amounted to a serious and wide-ranging attempt to tighten immigration controls yet again. Central to this package was what became the 1996 Asylum and Immigration Act.

Despite extensive criticism and campaigning, the 1996 Act became law. It entailed a number of new measures, one of which was to have the most serious and long-lasting impact on local authorities: the removal of entitlement to all social security benefits and local authority housing provision from 'in-country asylum seekers' and those appealing against the refusal of a claim. What was often not realised was that those who lost entitlement to cash benefit also lost entitlement to a range of welfare provision which depended on being a benefit claimant, such as educational grants, free school meals, free dentistry and eye care.

From October 1996 everybody who became subject to immigration control (including port asylum seekers) was barred from claiming Child Benefit, Family Credit, Disability Living Allowance, Disability Working Allowance, Severe Disablement Allowance or Attendance Allowance – although contributory benefits such as contributions-based Jobseeker's Allowance and pensions were not affected.

The exchange of information between local and central government officers and the Home Office, which had been proposed by the 'efficiency scrutiny', also went ahead. The Immigration and Nationality Department (IND) issued a circular to local authorities in October

1996, which invited them to use IND facilities to identify claimants who might be ineligible for a benefit or service because of their immigration status. It also encouraged local authorities to pass information to the IND about suspected immigration offenders. It was intended particularly for those administering the allocation of social housing, Housing Benefit, Council Tax Benefit and Student Awards. As the National Homeless Alliance explained:

> One of the main impacts of the Asylum and Immigration Act is the extension of immigration checks to housing allocations and to all homeless applications. If the Home Office learns that someone has received a public funds benefit, s/he may lose her/his right to stay in the country, fail to get an extension to her/his permission to stay, or find that her/his conditions of staying in the UK are affected.
>
> (NHA 1998: 4)

The Greater Manchester Immigration Aid Unit summed up the political consequences of the connection between welfare entitlement and immigration status:

> Firstly it means that every black person is made accountable for their immigration status in claiming an entitlement. Secondly it means that applying for such welfare or social benefits could jeopardise immigration status and now be a criminal offence by being a recourse to public funds. Thirdly it means the supposed caring agencies of the state and their workers are transformed into immigration police.
>
> (Cohen 1996: 7)

The new role of local authorities

Once the Asylum Act had become law there were two major consequences. First, there were even higher levels of destitution amongst asylum seekers (Webber 1997). Second, the Act stimulated a number of legal challenges by organisations concerned with refugees and asylum. The challenges established that local authorities had a duty to provide support to asylum seekers under existing legislation – in particular the 1948 National Assistance Act (which it was assumed had been superseded by modern social security law) and the 1989 Children Act. Local authorities had acquired the responsibility for providing basic support (essentially accommodation and food) to destitute asylum seekers. However, government ruled that simply providing cash payments was unlawful. Support under the National Assistance Act, which was to asylum seekers without children, had therefore to be 'in kind'.

Under the Children Act, there was much less room for argument about the duties of local authorities. Under Section 17 they had to 'safeguard and promote the welfare of children within their area who are in need; and . . . promote the upbringing of such children by their families, by providing a range and level of services appropriate to those children's needs . . . any service provided by an authority in the exercise of functions conferred on them by this section may be provided for the family of a particular child in need or for any member of his/her family . . .' Section 20 was more specific:

> Every local authority shall provide accommodation for any child in need within their area who appears to them to require accommodation as a result of . . . the person who has been caring for him/her being prevented (whether or not permanently, and for whatever reason) from providing him/her with suitable accommodation or care.
>
> (NHA 1998: 4)

Under the Children Act it was possible for local authorities to provide families with cash payments, thus avoiding some of the headaches created by the insistence that provision of services must be in kind under the National Assistance Act

Local authorities were now responsible for forms of support which would have been more appropriately managed through central government or through a reversion to welfare benefits. The Association of Directors of Social Services argued that: 'The current situation has all the defects of pre-welfare state provision, including variations from one authority to the next, and effective restrictions on the movement of people from one area to another' (ADSS 1997).

Under the 1996 Housing Act certain groups of 'persons from abroad' no longer qualified for homelessness assistance nor entry to an authority's register. Asylum seekers who were no longer entitled to benefits were not entitled to any help if homeless. Those who were entitled to benefits could be placed in temporary accommodation only. If they lost their benefits following a negative Home Office decision on their asylum claim they also lost entitlement to accommodation as homeless and could face eviction (NHA 1998).

However, under the National Assistance Act local authorities had a duty to provide accommodation – which often took the form of bed and breakfast accommodation. One crucial development was that a number of local authorities sought and won the right to 'export' asylum seekers to other parts of the country. These 'out of borough' placements have continued ever since and pioneered the dispersal of asylum seekers before it became government policy.

The negative impact of local authorities becoming responsible for destitute asylum seekers in the absence of state support, has been widely attested. One study of local authority officers responsible for homelessness (Rahilly 1998) found wide variations in provision and considerable uncertainty about eligibility. A major study about social housing for refugees and asylum seekers (Zetter and Pearl 1999) found that the Housing and Asylum Acts had created insurmountable barriers for asylum seekers, resulting in an unpredictable and chaotic situation, marginalisation and exclusion. In places, support workers reported 'shocking levels of basic unmet need, from shoes and clothes falling apart, to serious medical conditions going untreated' (Webber 1997: 75). According to one public health professional in East London:

> An audit of my own case histories in east London suggests that mental health problems are increasing at an alarming rate among asylum seekers. These are caused not by experience of traumatic events in their country of origin, nor by torture or pathology, but by chronic depression and dependencies created by grinding poverty, homelessness and mistreatment in the UK.
>
> (Savigar 1998)

How did a new Labour Government respond to this horror?

Labour: what kind of modernisation?

After a Labour Government came to office in 1997, it promised to modernise the whole immigration and asylum system. In 1998 it published the White Paper *Fairer, Faster and Firmer: a modern approach to immigration and asylum* (Home Office 1998). The call to combine firmness and fairness in immigration controls echoed the language of the previous Conservative Government. It gave the impression that there was no contradiction between these two elements and that striking a balance between them would be an essentially pragmatic task. This ignores the way in which immigration controls throughout the past century have grown out of, and in turn reinforced, the assumption that particular groups of 'foreigners' threaten to undermine the fabric of the nation and grab a share of its limited resources. This was the justification used by the Conservatives for their legislation and the publication of the White Paper made it clear that the same fundamental assumptions were driving Labour's plans. Hence the concern to distinguish between 'genuine' refugees and those whom officialdom now calls 'abusive' rather than 'bogus' asylum seekers. This was a modernisation of immigration legislation, not in the sense that it broke with the past to establish something new, but in the sense that it attempted to be more systematic in the application and extension of both external and internal controls.

When it came to translating its modern approach into specific policies, the White Paper made it clear that Labour would not repeal previous Conservative legislation but would strengthen and extend it (see Mynott 1999).

On coming to office, Labour had recognised that the system of supporting asylum seekers which they had inherited was 'a shambles' (Home Office 1998: ii). Their response, however, was to move towards an even more draconian system which generalised the worst aspects of the old arrangements, especially the principle of providing support in kind. The distinction between 'port' and 'in-country' asylum seekers was to be abolished – but not by restoring the rights of every asylum seeker to social security benefits and housing. Instead, the right to claim benefits was to be removed from *all* asylum seekers. The justification for this was that:

> Cash based support is administratively convenient and usually though not inevitably less expensive in terms of unit cost. Provision in kind is more cumbersome to administer, but experience has shown that this is less attractive and provides less of a financial inducement for those who would be drawn by a cash scheme.
>
> (Home Office 1998: 39)

The government made it clear that it was prepared to pick and mix the worst aspects of other European Union states' asylum policies. As the Campaign Against Racism and Fascism put it: 'Most European countries now have an asylum reception system involving a degree of compulsion, or a voucher system: Britain has gone for both, for about the harshest possible option for those who need support' (CARF 1999). Labour's asylum policy generalised the worst practices found across the EU *and* the worst aspects of the existing asylum system developed by the Conservatives. The policy has three main aspects: increased detention and deportation (which is unfortunately outside the scope of this chapter); the introduction of vouchers; and forced dispersal to regions outside London and the south-east of England.

Under the new system, the responsibility for issuing vouchers and organising the dispersal of asylum seekers has been taken over by a new agency, the National Asylum Support Service (NASS), which is part of the Immigration and Nationality Directorate of the Home Office. To those who have come into contact with it, the most obvious characteristics of NASS have been its bungling incompetence, lack of accountability and its punitive decisions. Equally noteworthy, however, is the fact that responsibility for organising social support for asylum seekers has now been shifted entirely away from the Department of Social Security and into the Home Office, the department of state which is also responsible for enforcement of immigration control. This brings the UK into line with practice in most other EU States (UNHCR 2000). This does not mean that local authorities or the voluntary sector no longer play any role in the provision of support. Rather, they operate under the aegis of NASS and its centrally determined policy and procedures. NASS has responsibility for co-ordinating the voucher scheme and the forced dispersal policy. Across Britain, 13 regional consortia were set up, which were led by local authorities, but were supposed to include other statutory and voluntary sector bodies. Since NASS became the responsible authority it has signed contracts with many of the regional consortia to provide accommodation – but it has signed more contracts with private landlords.

Introduction of vouchers

Having decided to generalise the principle of cashless support to all new asylum seekers, Labour illustrated its infatuation with the private sector by awarding the operation of the voucher scheme to a multi-national company, Sodexho. In its attempt to encourage large retailers and supermarkets to sign up to the scheme, Sodexho notoriously boasted of the government rule which forbade shops from giving change when vouchers were used. It urged retailers: 'don't miss this revenue making opportunity' (Sodexho Pass nd).

The voucher scheme has received more publicity and caused more revulsion than any other aspect of Labour's new asylum system. Its deliberate stigmatisation of asylum seekers is an open invitation to racist discrimination against them. Transport and General Workers Union (TGWU) General Secretary, Bill Morris argued that Home Office policies on asylum had 'given life to the racists' and called for the scrapping of the 'degrading and inhuman' asylum voucher scheme (*Independent*, 15 April 2000). This demand was taken up by the TUC, and threatened to win the support of delegates at Labour's 2000 Annual

Conference. In order to avoid losing the vote, Labour's leadership promised a 'comprehensive review of the asylum support system'. The government's betrayal was swift. By November it transpired that the 'comprehensive review' was to be an 'operational' not a 'policy' review, carried out by immigration minister, Barbara Roche, with a clear preference to simply provide vouchers in smaller denominations. Morris declared himself 'utterly disillusioned', but insisted that 'vouchers are an affront to human dignity on which my union will not compromise' (*Independent*, 23 November 2000).

Despite the restricted scope of the government review, the TGWU, together with Oxfam and the Refugee Council, submitted a report drawing on the experiences of fifty organisations working with asylum seekers across the UK. The summary of its findings illustrated the appalling impact of the voucher scheme:

- All 50 organisations agree that since the introduction of the voucher scheme they have seen an increase in the number of asylum seekers experiencing problems.
- 35 organisations (70 per cent) say that they have seen cases of asylum seekers experiencing hunger.
- 41 organisations (82 per cent) say asylum seekers are not able to buy enough food.
- 48 organisations (96 per cent) say asylum seekers are not able to buy other essential items.
- 49 out of the 50 organisations (98 per cent) feel that asylum seekers cannot maintain good health under the voucher scheme.
- 35 organisations (70 per cent) have experience of dealing with asylum seekers on vouchers suffering from anxiety or mental health problems.
- 35 organisations (70 per cent) say that asylum seekers have complained to them of poor treatment from shops accepting vouchers.
- 32 organisations (64 per cent) have seen asylum seekers suffering because of delay or non-arrival of vouchers.
- 31 organisations (62 per cent) have seen asylum seekers who complain about hostility from other shoppers.
- 27 organisations (54 per cent) have seen asylum seekers who complain that shops are inventing additional restrictions on the use of vouchers.
- 49 of the 50 organisations (98 per cent) state that the voucher scheme is creating serious difficulties.
- 46 organisations (92 per cent) say that asylum seekers are not coping well with the voucher scheme.

- 46 organisations (92 per cent) state that asylum seekers are unable to keep in touch with their lawyer.
- 49 say that their organisation had found it harder to help people to resolve their problems.
- 39 organisations (78 per cent) say that they had not been able to liaise effectively with the new administrative structures on behalf of clients.
- 38 organisations (76 per cent) state that they now have less time to work with refugees who have been granted refugee status or exceptional leave to remain.
- 41 organisations (82 per cent) state that they have incurred additional expenses as a result of the introduction of the voucher scheme.
- 47 organisations (94 per cent) say they had received complaints from asylum seekers about being unable to travel.
- 42 organisations (84 per cent) say that they have seen cases of asylum seekers who have lost some of the value of their vouchers through not receiving change, or who had made unnecessary purchases in order to avoid losing change.

(Oxfam /TGWU/Refugee Council 2000)

The major recommendations of the report were the introduction of a cash-based system of support with access to Income-Support-related benefits; the immediate provision of change on vouchers; and a campaign by government to improve public understanding of basic facts about asylum seekers. (The result of the review was not available at the time of writing.)

Yet while the voucher system has rightly received widespread condemnation from all those seeking to defend asylum seekers, the response to the forced dispersal policy has been somewhat more ambivalent. This was well expressed in comments by Chief Executive of the Kings Fund, Rabbi Julia Neuberger, in the introduction to the Oxfam/TGWU/Refugee Council report: 'The voucher system should be abolished at once, and replaced with cash entitlements for all asylum seekers. The dispersal system should be more in tune with the ability of communities to support new arrivals' (Oxfam/TGWU/Refugee Council 2000: 4). In other words, the voucher scheme had to go, but the dispersal scheme might be reformable.

Forced dispersal

From 2000, asylum seekers became the responsibility of the National Asylum Support Service. Asylum seekers are now forcibly dispersed to areas outside of London, regardless of any family, friends or specialist support which is more often available to them in the capital. If they refuse to go, they are deemed to have forfeited any right to accommodation.

The plan was that NASS would contract with regional consortia led by local authorities, and including the private sector and the voluntary sector, to provide accommodation and subsistence to destitute asylum seekers. Support would be 'offered as a last resort to those who have no other means including support from relatives and friends to which they can turn' (Home Office 1998: 38). They would get no choice over the type of accommodation they were to be placed in, nor the area to which they would be sent. One offer would be made and any refusal by the asylum seeker would mean the withdrawal of any right to accommodation. Asylum seekers would, however, be allowed to apply for vouchers without applying for accommodation.

Crucial to whether forced dispersal would succeed was the co-operation of local authorities and the Local Government Association (LGA), the umbrella organisation representing all local authorities in England and Wales. The LGA was 'very concerned about the use of vouchers, which evidence from local authorities with current problems shows can be costly, bureaucratic and stigmatising' (Oxfam/TGWU/Refugee Council 2000: 1). Yet when it came to the question of accommodation, the LGA was a willing and leading partner in helping government to organise forced dispersal to regions outside London:

> The LGA supports a national approach to the national responsibility towards asylum seekers imposed by the Geneva Convention. The proposals in the Bill will remove the intolerable burden currently placed upon a small number of local authorities for asylum seeker support, and allow for the development of strategic approaches to the placement, support and settlement of asylum seekers and refugees.
> Whilst we support a national approach, we wish to emphasise that the fair and effective delivery of the proposals will rely upon local services, experience and knowledge – it will be important to avoid the imposition of centrally determined arrangements.
> (LGA 1999)

The position of the Association of London Government (an umbrella organisation for the London borough councils) was even more supportive of the government's plans: 'Subject to robust arrangements, that will properly refer destitute asylum seekers and secure adequate support, the new arrangements offer a considerable improvement on the current position' (ALG 1998).

There are several criticisms which can be made of the stance taken by local authorities. First and foremost, despite the increase in the number of asylum claims in the 1990s, it is not the number of asylum seekers as such which is the cause of problems to local authorities, but the discriminatory policies relating to their reception and support. With the London Research Council estimating that 85 per cent of refugees and asylum seekers (240 000–280 000) in the UK were living in London in 1997 (Audit Commission 2000a: 2), it would be wrong to claim that local authorities have not experienced pressures. However, it is necessary to be precise about exactly what those pressures are and what causes them.

In terms of housing, the major problem is a shortage of *affordable temporary* housing. This is because, as the Audit Commission has pointed out: 'Councils have to use temporary accommodation to meet their housing responsibilities for both in-country and port applicants because permanent accommodation cannot be offered to asylum seeking households until their immigration status is resolved' (Audit Commission 2000a: 8). In the context of a general problem of homelessness, there are two main consequences of this enforced use of temporary accommodation: poor-quality accommodation continues to be used and private landlords drive up the rents they charge. Even in the case of those asylum seekers who retained the right to social security benefits (as port asylum seekers did after the 1996 legislation), local authorities still bore charges to their general funds because of the way housing benefit rates are calculated: 'Fixed ceilings for housing benefits – tied to a multiple of average council dwelling rents – may be lower than prevailing private sector rents or room charges, leaving the local authority to find the difference' (Audit Commission 2000b: 12).

More fundamentally, there is not a shortage of housing as such in London, but of affordable, good-quality housing. Serious difficulties are faced by low-paid (and not-so-low-paid) public sector workers who are priced out of the housing market of London, the Home Counties and the south-east. This has been compounded by a shortage of social housing provided by housing associations, the transfer of much existing council housing into private hands and the virtual abandonment of new building of council properties. Housing is of course still being built, but for the profit of housebuilders and sometimes of buyers too:

> [L]arge numbers of the houses built ostensibly to solve Britain's urgent housing crisis have instead been sold abroad as speculative investments. In 1997, a remarkable 50 per cent of all the new homes built in Central and Inner London were purchased in the Far East.

Domestic demand is also strong. There are 224 000 second homes in Britain, which is, coincidentally, roughly equivalent to the official number of homeless families and single people.

(Monbiot 2000: 157)

The plight of asylum seekers forced to live in substandard accommodation is simply the most extreme expression of a general housing crisis, at its most acute in London, created by the free market. Yet rather than reexamine the free market policies which create this housing crisis, the Labour government proposed the forced dispersal of asylum seekers – which, incidentally, does nothing to solve the housing crisis.

Additionally, when authorities in London and the south-east talked of an 'intolerable burden', and the Labour Government justified itself by the need to ease the pressure on London and Kent councils, they were accommodating to the discourse which presents asylum seekers as competitors for a naturally fixed level of resources. Such an attitude has always fed hostility to immigrants and, prompted by right-wing political forces, can harden into racism. This is particularly likely to happen when a group such as asylum seekers, who are incessantly demonised by large sections of the British Press, are officially deemed problematic and in need of dispersal around the country. The ground is perfectly prepared for any racists within the receiving areas to demand 'no asylum seekers here'.

There was always a far better and simpler alternative available. The perfectly correct adoption of a national approach to a national responsibility did not have to entail the adoption of dispersal and vouchers. The most obvious solution would be to allow asylum seekers the right to access housing, Income Support and related social security benefits in the same way as British citizens, recognised refugees or those granted Exceptional Leave to Remain. Local authorities could have taken up this call, while lobbying or campaigning for any increased central funding necessary to provide services specifically required by asylum seekers (such as translation, for example) or to expand general services used by a local population of which asylum seekers are part. This would deal with the problem of local authorities taking on those responsibilities which would be more appropriately discharged by national government, and which the authorities are not fully reimbursed for.

The results of dispersal

As predicted by opponents of the 1999 Immigration and Asylum Act, the dispersal scheme has worsened the conditions in which asylum seekers are forced to live. There is evidence of many people refusing to be dispersed at all (Audit Commission 2000a: 3) and others returning to London, 'disappearing' from the authorities if they have to. As if it were not bad enough to be arbitrarily separated from friends, family and others of the same nationality, asylum seekers continued to be dumped in sometimes appalling accommodation.

Shelter, the charity which campaigns with homeless and badly housed people, inspected 154 dwellings in London and three other cities occupied by asylum seekers in the first three months of 2000, just before NASS came into operation. It reported that nearly a fifth were unfit for human habitation, 19 per cent were infested, 28 per cent were overcrowded and 83 per cent were exposed to unacceptable risks of fire: 'Shelter has found that often people who are already very vulnerable and frightened are being placed in housing with appalling standards in the private rented sector. Its investigation shows that agencies have placed many in dangerous, overcrowded and extremely poor quality accommodation' (Garvie 2001).

Shelter also pointed out that unlike most other private tenants, asylum seekers housed via NASS have no legal protection from eviction, and that NASS's complaints procedure requires tenants to register complaints with the accommodation provider. Combined with a fear of authority, an unwillingness to be seen as ungrateful, and language problems, it is no wonder that, despite sometimes appalling accommodation, so few complain. Shelter argued that the legislation of 1993, 1996 and 1999 had led to a serious deterioration of housing conditions for asylum seekers, and the return of the spectre of Rachmanite landlords growing rich on contracts to house asylum seekers:

> The cumulative impact of legislative changes has been to remove choice and autonomy for homeless asylum seekers. Instead, they have become dependent on a bureaucratic framework which allocates them housing without giving them the opportunity to express a preference. . . . A significant proportion of placements, regardless of route are now likely to be in the private rented sector . . . [which] includes much of the worst managed, most unsafe and dangerous housing available. . . . The concern was that it would be this group of landlords who would become involved in housing asylum seekers: that a group of people with far fewer rights would become a tempting new market for the worst landlords.
>
> (Garvie 2001: 6–10)

In autumn 2000, Manchester City Council provided evidence of the state of private sector accommodation to which NASS had dispersed asylum seekers. It investigated claims of private landlords attempting to classify unrelated single adults as 'families' to flout rules governing multi-occupancy and cram more people into houses; buying up low-value property in the belief that through accommodating asylum seekers they would recoup the outlay within a short period; private providers proposing to double and even treble the number of people housed in hostel-type accommodation; and vulnerable people left without support or information on local community and health services (*Manchester Evening News* 22 September 2000). Of 42 properties subsequently inspected, 14 were found to be unfit for human habitation and a further 20 were in a state of serious disrepair (DeSouza 2000).

In theory, the Home Office had planned to send people to 'cluster zones' which were 'multi-ethnic' (thus supposedly reducing the likelihood of racist attack) and could provide services for particular nationalities and languages. In practice, dispersal has been to the poorest areas with high levels of empty housing stock. In its cynical disregard for the well-being of asylum seekers, the Home Office has commissioned accommodation from private landlords at rock-bottom prices. The government has refused to disclose precisely how much NASS is paying each company, because the information is commercially sensitive. The Home Office has also driven down the price it is prepared to pay to the regional consortia of local authorities, which are organising the reception of dispersed asylum seekers. Indeed the South West Consortium reported an admission by Barbara Roche that: 'Price is the main driver in arranging accommodation for asylum seekers' (South West Consortium for Asylum Seekers 2000).

Manchester City Councillors, involved in the North West Consortium reported that after months of talks about signing a contract with NASS: 'When we sat down to finalise it they introduced three new requirements that were all aimed at driving down costs in a way that we thought was unjustified' (*Manchester Evening News* 22 September 2000). After eventually signing the contract, one Council officer concluded: 'I have never come across an agency which seems so intent on badly treating asylum seekers' (DeSouza 2000).

In September 2000, Liverpool City Council withdrew from the North West consortium after NASS sent 1000 asylum seekers to private landlords in Liverpool, while refusing to pay costs of £170 000 which the Council claimed it had already incurred accommodating dispersed asylum seekers (*Daily Telegraph* 21 September 2000). In April 2000 NASS had signed a contract with Landmark Liverpool to house more than 600 asylum seekers in two 15-storey blocks abandoned by Liverpool City Council as unfit for their own tenants. Another company, Clearsprings, abandoned nearly 100 asylum seekers from a dozen nationalities in Nelson, Lancashire, without telling the health authority or the local council of their presence (*Observer* 28 May 2000). In their report into the situation in Scotland, Save the Children and the Scottish Refugee Council found racism and appalling living conditions:

> Children and young people dispersed to Scotland are being located in socially disadvantaged areas in which they experience problems associated with property maintenance, vandalism, lack of places to play, limited social services, harassment, etc, all of which are compounded by their negative and differential status in the local community.
>
> (Macaskill and Petrie 2000: 7)

Nor was racism confined to Scotland. There is no doubt that dispersal has been accompanied by a high level of racism, fed by an often hostile local Press. According to the Audit Commission, of 161 local Press articles they analysed in October/November 1999, only six per cent cited the positive contribution made by asylum seekers and refugees (Audit Commission 2000a: 33). Roma organisations have reported 'a whole list of cases of children being threatened at northern schools, forcing their parents to return to London' (Bright and Ahmed 2000). According to one activist from the North East Coalition for Asylum Rights: 'asylum seekers have been the target of racist abuse and attacks. Many feel under siege. The British National Party have been leafleting and now have the confidence to stand candidates in local elections on an anti-asylum seekers platform, given succour by the racist language of politicians and the tabloid press' (Anon 2001). A spokesperson for an organisation working with asylum seekers argued: 'We see a fair number who have experienced racial attacks, and a lot of it is to do with people being dispersed into areas of cities where you would not necessarily want to put them. Some people are being sent into areas of Liverpool and other places where you just don't go if you have a black face, yet people are being dispersed to those areas and almost inevitability there have been race attacks on them' (Goldman 2001).

How far some districts truly are no-go areas for black people may be debatable. In most areas a constant battle takes place between racist ideas and actions, and anti-racist responses. What is true is that it is to areas with pockets of serious racism that asylum seekers have often been dispersed to face hostility. Even the Association of Chief Police Officers has concluded that 'ill-informed, adverse media coverage' of asylum seekers has contributed to a rise in racial tension and increased risk of public disorder. 'Racist expressions towards asylum seekers appear to have become common currency and acceptable in a way which would never be tolerated towards any other minority' (*Guardian* 23 January 2001).

Even in areas to which only tiny numbers of asylum seekers had been dispersed by the end of 2000, some thought that the high-profile political hostility to asylum seekers had led to an increase in racism (which proves again that it is not numbers as such, but politics and racism which are crucial). When Jan Martin Passelbessi was murdered in Newport, South Wales in June 2000, the head of the Wales Commission for Racial Equality argued that the 150 per cent increase in racist incidents reported to the police since November 1999 was due to adverse publicity given to asylum seekers being dispersed to Wales and a lack of knowledge about the numbers involved: 'the people who are really suffering are, in fact, black and ethnic minorities who have enjoyed a long period of peacefulness here and are now being victimised' (*Guardian* 16 June 2000).

In June 2000, soon after dispersal began, the Audit Commission had reported on arrangements for the dispersal of asylum seekers. While the report accepted the government's reading of the situation and stated its main aim was 'to help local agencies to make the policy of dispersal work' it did point out that: 'Without effective support, asylum seekers could easily become locked in a cycle of exclusion and dependency in their new community. Alternatively, they could simply "vote with their feet" and return to London, again putting pressure on health and education services in the capital' (Audit Commission 2000a: 4).

By the end of 2000 this is precisely what appears to have happened. *The Observer* reported that the dispersal system was in disarray: 'Local councils and refugee groups have warned Ministers that asylum seekers in their thousands are drifting back to London after dispersal, or are simply choosing to remain in the capital or South East without any money for housing.' Refugee Council Chief Executive, Nick Hardwick, said that asylum seekers were rejecting dispersal in droves because they were often sent to sink estates where they were too frightened to venture outside their homes (*Observer* 31 December 2000).

In early 2001, it was reported by organisations contracted to look after asylum seekers, that families and friends were being arbitrarily split up and sent to towns in different parts of the country; families who did not speak English were being sent to places and left waiting at bus stations for hours because no one came to meet them; people were being dispersed to estates where it is known that racial attacks were likely; there was large-scale failure to ensure that the vouchers (the asylum seekers' only source of income) actually got through on time to the needy families. 'So bad has been the treatment of many people that a picture of systematic failure bordering on abuse is disclosed' (Goldman 2001).

So all the talk of 'cluster zones' and 'multi-ethnic communities' by the government turned out to be diversionary window-dressing for the dumping of vulnerable people, often without any support whatsoever. Perhaps the most obvious point to make is that the removal of asylum seekers from mainstream welfare provision and the creation of an apartheid system using dispersal and vouchers has failed utterly in its own terms. It has had no impact whatsoever in deterring people from seeking asylum in the UK. Indeed, the figures for those seeking asylum in the UK rose to their highest ever level in 2000 (76 000). Compare this with the early 1990s when asylum seekers had virtually unrestricted access to mainstream social security and housing – and the numbers seeking asylum were many times smaller. The only conclusion to be drawn is that people move because they have to, not because they are attracted by generous cash benefits. Yet in the topsy-turvy world of the immigration debate, right-wing newspapers conclude that Britain is a 'soft touch' and the ground is prepared for government ministers to pre-pare another turn of the screw.

Instead of restoring asylum seekers' right to claim social security benefits and giving them the right to work – which would be right *and* cheaper – Labour has created a new apartheid social security system, separate from and deliberately inferior to the already miserable levels of the welfare state. It would be difficult to deliberately engineer conditions more likely to promote racist attacks.

Conclusion

Such is the huge amount of misrepresentation of migrants that any-thing which highlights the terrible conditions suffered by asylum seekers, or their true motivations, is worthwhile and valuable. However, specialist reports and voluntary organisations too often give the impres-sion that the mistreatment of asylum seekers which takes place is an accidental outcome of policy; a mistake or an oversight, which will be rectified when people of good will point out the problem. The truth is somewhat harsher. The mistreatment of asylum seekers and others sub-ject to immigration control is deliberate.

Faced with this reality, we are not about to see local authorities act as tribunes of the exploited and oppressed. There have been times in the past when local councils have done so. We need only think of George Lansbury and Poplar Labour Council in the 1920s (Branson 1979). In the 1980s Labour Party left-wingers saw 'municipal socialism' as a way to oppose the Thatcherism of the national government. The strategy eventually failed and its memory is reviled by New Labour. Yet, whatever its shortcomings, it was at least an attempt to defend the interests of working class people and to fight against racism. Moreover, there remains a public resonance for the attempt to use local government in this way. This can be seen by the election of one of the most famous figures associated with municipal socialism, former Greater London Council leader, Ken Livingstone, as Mayor of London in May 2000.

Today's Labour-run local councils are not about to lead any resistance. It will be down to campaigning bodies and asylum seekers themselves (notwithstanding the severe difficulties for this group in organising themselves) to argue for forced dispersal and the voucher system to be scrapped. Within such campaigns, those who oppose immigration controls for all the reasons outlined in this book, need to generalise from the experience of the struggles which are mounted, attempting to win wider numbers of people to understand the pernicious role of immigration controls in institutionalising racism, punishing immigrants and undermining the struggle for working class unity.

At the same time it is important for those activists operating in the regions to which asylum seekers have been dispersed to be tactically adept. They must locate their arguments within a clear defence of asylum seekers. To simply say 'no to dispersal' without first having said 'asylum seekers are welcome in our city' would be to risk echoing the racists who are opposed to dispersal because they are opposed to the arrival of asylum seekers, full stop. Activists, through their campaigns, need to create a political pole of attraction to which are drawn anti-racists, asylum seekers and all those who oppose scapegoating – whether their motivation is that of a basic humanitarianism, anti-imperialism, a desire to forge working class unity or whatever.

Part of this campaign should be to approach local Labour-run councils and ask them to be part of a public defence of asylum seekers. Campaigners could encourage the council to publicise any positive aspects of its work – for example, highlighting attempts to tackle the horrendous conditions of many properties owned by private landlords who have contracted with NASS to receive dispersed asylum seekers. Naturally, because local councils have been integral to dispersal, and because they may be fearful of electoral consequences, this approach would not be without its tensions. Council leaderships may well refuse

124   *Ed Mynott*

to become involved. But the proposal should still be put. If councils will not become part of a broad anti-racist defence of asylum seekers, independently organised campaigners will mount it anyway. If they agree, for example, to send out a clear message that 'asylum seekers are welcome in our city' this can give much greater confidence to anti-racists in that city. That remains true even if campaigners subsequently come into conflict with the council over its collaboration with national government in implementing policies such as dispersal, which are not about supporting asylum seekers properly but making their lives even more miserable than before.

References

ADSS (1997) *Asylum Seekers Briefing*, London: Association of Directors of Social Services, April.

ALG (1998) *Refugees and Asylum Seekers* (*Report by Social Policy Officer to Leaders Committee*) London: Association of London Government.

Anon (2001) 'NASS (Nasty, Arrogant, Stupid Service)' *National Coalition of Anti Deportation Campaigns Newsletter*, 21 (January–March).

Audit Commission (2000a) *Another Country*: *implementing dispersal under the Immigration and Asylum Act 1999*, London: Audit Commission.

——(2000b) *A New City*: *supporting asylum seekers and refugees in London* (Briefing), London: Audit Commission.

Branson, N. (1979) *Poplarism, 1919–1925*: *George Lansbury and the councillors revolt*, London: Lawrence and Wishart.

Bright, M. and Ahmed, K. (2000) 'Nowhere left to run to' *The Observer* 31 December.

Brown, R. (1995) 'Racism and immigration in Britain', *International Socialism* 68 (Autumn): 3–35.

CARF (1999) 'Exclusion: New Labour style' *Campaign against Racism and Fascism*, 49 (April/May).

Cohen, S. (1996) *Another Brick in the Wall*, Manchester: Greater Manchester Immigration Aid Unit.

DeSouza, E. (2000) Speech at 'Asylum Seekers in Manchester' Conference, 23 November 2000.

Garvie, D. (2001) *Far from Home*: *the housing of asylum seekers in private rented accommodation* (Media briefing), London: Shelter.

Goldman, T. (2001) 'NASS which disperses asylum seekers is also abusing them' *National Coalition of Anti Deportation Campaigns Newsletter*, 21 (January–March).

Home Office (1998) *Fairer, Faster, Firmer*: *a modern approach to immigration and asylum*, London: The Stationery Office.

LGA (1999) *Immigration and Asylum Bill*: *written submission to Commons Special Standing Committee* (Briefing paper), London: Local Government Association.

Macaskill, S. and Petrie, M. (2000) *I Didn't Come Here for Fun: listening to the views of children and young people who are refugees or asylum seekers in Scotland*, Edinburgh: Save the Children.

Monbiot, G. (2000) *Captive State: The corporate takeover of Britain*, London: Macmillan.

Mynott, E. (1999) *Immigration, Asylum and the Provision of Services in Manchester: a preliminary report*, Manchester: Manchester Metropolitan University.

NACAB (1996) *Failing the Test: Citizens Advice Bureaux clients' experience of the habitual residence test in social security*, London: National Association of Citizens Advice Bureaux.

NHA (1998) *Asylum Seekers' Rights* (Briefing), London: National Homeless Alliance.

Oxfam/TGWU/Refugee Council (2000) *Token Gestures: the effects of the voucher scheme on asylum seekers and organisations in the UK*, London: Oxfam.

Rahilly, S. (1998) 'Housing for the homeless and immigration control: the provisions of the Housing Act and the Asylum and Immigration Act 1996', *Journal of Social Welfare and Family Law* 20, (3).

Savigar, S. (1998) 'Double trouble', *Nursing Times*, 16 September, 94(37).

Sodexho Pass (nd) *Asylum Seekers Voucher System* (Sodexho Pass document for retailers).

South West Consortium for Asylum Seekers (2000) *Newsletter*, No.5, 3 October.

TUC (1995) *Race and Social Security*, London: Trades Union Congress.

UNHCR (2000) *Reception Standards for Asylum Seekers in the European Union*, Geneva: United Nations High Commission for Refugees.

Webber, F. (1997) 'Asylum seekers: caught by the Act', *Race and Class*, 38(3): 73–74.

Zetter, R. and Pearl, M. (1999) *Managing to Survive: refugees, asylum seekers and housing management in registered social landlords*, London: Policy Press.

8 From welfare to authoritarianism

The role of social work in immigration controls

Beth Humphries

Introduction

Welfare has always been a site of struggle in discourses about, and allocation of resources in relation to, issues of class, race and gender. Immigration policy is a particularly fruitful area for illustrating the ways in which health, education, housing, social services and the whole gamut of benefits related to income support, have been used to define the boundaries of nation, and for purposes of inclusion and exclusion (see Hayes 2000; and Chapters 3 and 10 of this volume). This chapter focuses on social work, an activity that in the recent past has been extraordinarily explicit in its stand on anti-racist and anti-discriminatory practice, but which has been at times rather naïve about its contradictory positioning, and which latterly has been increasingly drawn into a disciplinary and surveillance role in policing the poor, to the extent of having now been 'tamed' (Jones and Novak 1999). The chapter describes some of the ways this has taken place and, in the wake of the 1996 and 1999 immigration legislation, it will examine moves by the Home Office towards enlisting the co-operation of welfare professionals in identifying and excluding those not entitled to services. It will also consider the implications for people subject to immigration controls.

The contradictory role of social work

The link between welfare and exclusion has been well documented (see Cohen 1996; Taylor 1996). Ever since the foundations of the welfare state were laid, a recurring theme in housing, education, health and income support policies has been one of exclusivity. There has never been a time when welfare professionals have not been involved in remoralising the poor, in identifying those undeserving or not entitled to a service, and in policing the boundaries of welfare (Hayes 2000). It should not come as a surprise therefore, that they are also being enlisted by the Home Office in the internal control of immigration. Chris Jones's (1983) historical analysis of the development of social work shows how social work as an institution has to be considered as one of the agencies of class control and regulation in Britain. One might also draw attention to its regulatory role in confirming normative relationships involving gender and 'race'. Jones is careful not to argue that this is an unambiguous role, and indeed sees possibilities to resist and subvert its prevailing intent, and to challenge ideologies designed to control the poor.

The dominant discourses defining social work since the 1940s and in the context of 'welfarism', have assumed a benign if paternalistic relationship, where problems could be solved through a therapeutic relationship involving casework with individual families. Its knowledge was derived predominantly from psychodynamic theory and ego-psychology and provided a legitimation for social work to locate itself within the 'psy' professions (Parton 1996a). As Parton (1996a: 9) says, the essential ambiguities, tensions and uncertainties that lay at the core of its operations remained partially submerged. Nevertheless, social workers have always been difficult employees. There has always been a recognition of and resistance to the oppressive role, and there have been times when resistance has resulted in direct conflict with the state (Bailey and Brake 1975; Parton 1996b).

With the neo-liberal approach of the Thatcher years, the rhetoric about the therapeutic and supportive role of social work changed to become more explicit about its controlling function through a greater emphasis on 'identifying risk' and on the bureaucratisation and managerial control of social work. After a brief attempt during the early 1990s to name and challenge structured oppression, professional training and behaviour has been regulated and compliance achieved with political and economic objectives through discourses of managerialism and 'competence', and a diluted version of 'anti-discriminatory practice' (Webb 1996). This taming process is designed to make social workers predictable, reliable state agents. During the 1980s and 1990s social workers, along with teachers, probation officers, youth workers and the educators of these groups, endured a sustained attack on their competence, their motives and their political agendas, and were portrayed as undermining British culture and 'the family'. The concept of 'political correctness' was introduced into the national vocabulary as a term of abuse towards these welfare professionals (see Jones 1993; Humphries 1997), and resulted in changes to their prescribed role and professional training which curtailed their autonomy and introduced tighter controls which worked against the interests of their clients. As Jones and Novak comment:

> In true materialist fashion, government from the mid-1980s onwards embarked upon a wholesale reorganisation of professional practice and training that would transform the nature of state welfare activity and lead to a routing of the welfare professions as a potential countervailing force.
>
> (Jones and Novak 1999: 158)

Work with children and their families, formerly focused on support and prevention, saw a major paradigm shift from 'child welfare' to 'child protection', characterised by a preoccupation with procedures and guidelines and away from the welfare-oriented approach of an earlier period (Otway 1996). Official policy has developed an obsession with 'risk' (Department of Health 1988; 1991; Social Services Inspectorate 1993), and training for social workers has progressively focused on identifying 'high-risk' situations. However as we shall see, the preoccupation with protecting children at risk does not appear to extend to children subject to immigration controls. The defining concept in the contemporary role of social work is 'control' rather than 'protection'.

The 1990 National Health Service and Community Care Act shifted the social work role from providers of care to assessors of need within restricted budgets, and purchasers of services from the voluntary and private sectors. But Parton (1996b) argues that the notion of 'risk' related to old people, disabled people and those with mental health problems or learning disabilities, is also of central concern in the implementation of the legislation and in the preoccupations of government. The role of the Probation Service was very clearly shifted from social casework to the more pragmatic role of dealing with high-risk offenders, underscored by its removal from any identification with social work. The arrival of a New Labour Government has brought with it a new authoritarianism, as illustrated in for example the current White Paper on mental health, which proposes to target and confine people perceived to be a risk to the public, *before* they have committed an offence. If this is not troubling enough, the new act will also introduce compulsory treatment orders under which mentally ill people who have, for whatever reason stopped taking their drugs, may be hospitalised and forced to take the drugs by whatever means are deemed to be convenient (see Rayner 2001).

Social work and the Home Office

It will be clear that in many ways, a role for social workers in immigration controls is consistent with the modern definition of their job. Stereotypes of immigrants and asylum seekers emphasise their dangerousness in descriptions of them as violent, thieving, neglectful of children, a drain on state benefits and as stealing 'our' jobs (Harding 2000). This legitimates action by state officials to protect the nation's resources and to justify the commonsense belief that 'some controls are needed', both to protect Britain from aggressive foreigners and to limit numbers admitted to this overcrowded island.

The Conservative Government sought to enforce and reinforce this role in very specific ways. After the introduction of the 1996 Asylum and Immigration and Appeals Act, the Home Office conducted what has become known as the 'efficiency scrutiny' on the enforcement of immigration laws, in order to ensure that no one should benefit from state provision who is not entitled to it (Hudson 1997). It was clear that agencies of welfare provision were viewed as an arm of the Home Office through their having been authorised to check the immigration and residence status of users. The scrutiny sought cooperation and partnership between the Home Office and the range of health, education and welfare services, in the checking of documentation and the general policing of provision. A press release issued on 13 October 1993 was headed *Home Secretary announces study of inter-agency cooperation on illegal immigration* and stated: 'the study will examine the efficiency of existing arrangements for cooperation between the Home Office's Immigration and Nationality Division and other key central and local government bodies. These include the police, agencies of the DSS, the Employment Service, the Health Service and housing authorities'. Although social services are not mentioned explicitly, the implication was that all statutory agencies would be included. Indeed a 'help line' was provided for any local authority workers who have concerns about anyone's immigration status, and training is given to assist in identifying offenders (Hayes 2000). The Home Secretary said in parliament that one of the purposes of close collaboration between the Home Office and the NHS and other welfare services was to strengthen immigration control, and to avoid the situation 'where illegal immigrants were able to escape detection because procedures for identifying them were unclear' (*Hansard*, 18 July 1995). This was emphasised again and again:

> Those here illegally can come into contact with many Government agencies. It is therefore sensible that we ensure that all of us are

making the most efficient use of the information available to us . . .
we should look afresh at ways in which Government as a whole –
central and local – could cooperate more effectively to prevent
abuse of the immigration laws and the drain on public funds which
it often represents.

(Michael Howard, reported in the *Guardian*, 9 May 1995)

During 1997, asylum teams were set up in social services departments to provide help to asylum seekers who, after the 1996 Act, were
no longer eligible for welfare benefits. Research was carried out by
Duvell and Jordan (2000) into teams in London, and reported that the
restrictions on the amount and form of help they were mandated to
provide meant that the teams were operating well below the standards
seen as acceptable for UK citizens: 'in other words, these social workers
were, by some criteria, violating human rights' (Jordan 2000: 140). The
researchers found that the study 'illustrated the fact that social workers
will volunteer to do the "dirty work" of social policy, even when this
involves intentional and systematic deprivation by official agencies, of
the means of dignified existence'. They resorted to stereotyping their
clients and to distancing themselves by defining clients' cultural practices in terms of problems and deficiencies, whilst at the same time
trying to protect the most vulnerable individuals from abuse by an
uncaring authority. Jordan concludes that the work of asylum teams
prefigured other aspects of New Labour policy developments in what
he calls 'enforcement counselling' (Jordan, 2000: 142) – systems for
replacing both cash benefit rights and social services, with in-kind provision, offering no options and giving officials complete power over
applicants.

Certainly the 1999 Immigration and Asylum Act – the third major
piece of immigration legislation of the 1990s – made clear that the New
Labour Government did not intend to backtrack on the trend set by
their predecessors. The new legislation is if anything, harsher than what
went before, particularly in the extension of the regulations to exclude
from benefits *all* those subject to immigration controls. The legislation
under which it had been possible to offer support – the National
Assistance Act 1948, the Health Services and Public Health Act 1968,
the National Health Service Act 1977, the Housing Act 1966 and section 17 of the Children Act 1989 – have all been amended to exclude not
only asylum seekers, but anyone caught in the net of immigration law.
Responsibility for their support has been taken over by a new national
agency under the Home Office, National Asylum Seekers Support
(NASS), which will contract with other agencies for services. Support is

'in kind', mainly through food vouchers. One offer of accommodation is made, with no choice as to the location, and anyone leaving the accommodation offered to them will lose the right to support. The result will surely be destitution, poverty, exploitation, ill health and sometimes death.

Policing social services

Some of those who are denied support have found their way to social services seeking help. The contradictions in the positioning of social workers are clear. Their professional values urge them to help wherever they can, yet they are asked to assess immigration status, on which that help is now dependent. They often have the resources to offer support and help, yet they are required to identify, exclude from services and report to the Home Office those who have been labelled 'illegal'. This is highly political behaviour and has ethical implications for professional workers. It raises moral questions about denying help to those who need it, and it risks collusion with the racist questioning of people with entitlement to the full benefits of welfare, specifically black British citizens. For if social workers are to check on immigration status before offering a service, *how do they know whom to question*? Research that has taken place in Manchester (Hayes 1995; Cohen *et al.* 1997; Jones 1998; Mynott 1999; Mynott and Humphries 2001) confirms the ambiguous and uncertain position in which local authorities find themselves. The research by Duvell and Jordan (2000) quoted earlier, and that undertaken by Mynott and Humphries (2001), give little hope that professional ethics will take precedence over organisational culture and policy. Indeed, as Jordan (2000: 142) comments, social workers are in the vanguard of public officials who negotiate with individuals over the terms and conditions of which services are given or refused – and asylum teams were the pioneers of this approach.

Care in the community, but not for all

The social work literature and social work research have had very little to say about the implications for the job brought about by the changes. However there are indications of a rather negative and punitive culture within local authorities, apparent in their attempts to restrict the legislation even further, in denying help to people in need of it. For example, overstayers, illegal entrants, those with leave to remain, but with a condition of no recourse to public funds, and those appealing against a decision, have no access to assistance if their need arises solely because of *the physical effects of actual or anticipated destitution.* This could be read to imply that there may be other grounds on which they might receive help. Recent cases considered by the Court of Appeal suggest that some local authorities interpret this as non-entitlement to a service on *any* grounds, and a reluctance to look for other reasons a person might require and be entitled to their help. The case of 'O' illustrates this attitude (Court of Appeal 2000). 'O' is a Nigerian woman who came to this country in 1989 and overstayed her leave. Her funds ran out in 1994, and a deportation order was made against her in 1996. She became ill, suffering from severe depression and multiple fibroids within her uterus. Her application for exceptional leave to remain (ELR) quoted the psychiatrist's report that if she returned to Nigeria, 'O' would not be able to obtain the required medication and her mental health would deteriorate rapidly. Her solicitor wrote to Wandsworth Council and asked for an assessment under the 1990 NHS and Community Care Act. The reply from Wandsworth's solicitor declined the request on the following grounds:

> As a matter of public policy a person cannot secure an advantage by way of reliance on his or her wrongdoing. ['O''s] application for assistance is a result of being unlawfully in this country. Your letter and the accompanying reports do not assert ['O'] is too ill to travel. In fact, it appears that in recent times she has been working as a child minder. It appears therefore that there are no factors outside ['O''s] control, which prevent her from leaving the UK.
>
> It is noted that you assert that if ['O'] returns to Nigeria there is a serious danger she would kill herself and/or be in conditions subjecting her to acute medical and physical suffering. However, in my Council's view, concerns about the quality of medical care in Nigeria and speculation about the possible consequences for ['O'] should she return there, are not sufficient grounds to render ['O'] eligible for assistance.
>
> (Court of Appeal 2000: 8)

These paragraphs contain all the classic assumptions and cynicism that the request is likely to be bogus and therefore inhumane treatment is justified. First, 'O' has acted illegally so she can be considered 'undeserving'; she is also likely to be feigning illness and lying about its seriousness (she is after all able to work as a baby sitter); she is not likely to die on the journey from the UK, and once she is out of the country we do not need to care what happens to her.

A similar narrow-mindedness was evident in the case of Mr Bhikha, a 60-year-old Kenyan who was granted six months leave as a visitor to the UK. He became ill with carcinoma of the duodenum and had to have radical surgery. He was refused leave to remain on health grounds and applied to Leicester City Council for assistance, as he was living a 'hand-to-mouth' existence and was homeless, living in mosques. Leicester refused help, again suggesting that he was not too ill to travel back to Kenya. In determining whether *destitution* was the sole cause of need (in which case 'O' and Mr Bhikha would not be entitled to help), the local authority might have taken account of other conditions that made their situation more acute, such as their illness, their age, any disability, as relevant in contributing to vulnerability. Clearly in both these cases, considerations of illegality took precedence over humanity. In making a judgment in favour of both these appellants, Lord Justice Brown recognised that returning home was not a real choice for either of them. He criticised the approach of the local authorities as 'applying (an) inflexible approach to a welfare scheme of last resort' (Court of Appeal 2000: 19), and went on to say:

> I would hold that the LA has no business with the applicant's immigration status save only for the purpose of learning why the care and attention 'is not otherwise available to them . . . it should be for the Home Office to decide . . . any claim for ELR . . . rather than for local authorities to, so to speak, starve immigrants out of the country by withholding last resort assistance from those who today will by definition be not merely destitute but for other reasons too, in urgent need of care and assistance.
>
> (Court of Appeal 2000: 20)

This judgment makes it clear that welfare assistance is about needs, not morality, although the Home Office – and the local authorities – appear to take a different view. As Lady Justice Hale pointed out in the same judgment (Court of Appeal 2000: 28), social workers are skilled at assessing need and arranging the appropriate services, as is their statutory duty under the Community Care Act 1990. They are not professionals in making moral judgements as between particular people with identical needs, nor are they skilled in assessing whether a person is subject to immigration control or has a real choice about whether or not to return to her/his home country. Immigration status is a complex matter, making the task of deciding on eligibility a questionable one. Yet the political climate that has been created encourages local authorities to attempt exactly that, both at the level of deciding on policy and at the level of individual social workers offering a service. One of the results of this is that social services departments are thrown into the arms of the Home Office in order to check immigration status before offering a service. In the study by Mynott and Humphries (2001), there was evidence that committees deciding on offering resources under Section 47 of the Children Act 1989, declined to offer support until the social worker making the application had checked status with the Home Office.

Children, social work and internal controls: a case of abuse and neglect

The scene is set for the treatment of children subject to immigration controls by the limit placed by the UK on its obligation under the 1951 Refugee Convention and other international treaties, to assist refugees. Specifically regarding children, the UK has entered a reservation about immigration control to the 1989 UN Convention on the Rights of the Child, refusing to be bound to ensure that a refugee child – or any child subject to immigration control – receives appropriate protection and humanitarian assistance:

> The reservation symbolises the relationship between immigration law and child law in the UK: it is one of the rare areas of UK law concerning children where the 'best interests principle' does not play a part or where the protection of the child is not the paramount concern.
>
> (Amnesty International 2000: 32)

The impact of this on some of the most vulnerable children in the world is one of systemic discrimination against them. Children in the UK legal system enjoy special protection, 'whether as parties in civil litigation, witnesses, the subjects of proceedings or indeed when charged with criminal offences' (Refugee Children's Consortium 2000: 2). 'Litigation friends' (previously *guardians ad litem*) are appointed for British children involved in civil proceedings. No such provision is made for asylum-seeking children, nor does the law guarantee the assistance of a legal representative. The government's document *Quality Protects* (Department of Health 1998) has set out a three-year programme to transform children's services, requiring local authorities to submit management action plans for meeting the objectives of the programme. A survey of all local authorities (Barnardo's 2000), found that none of those who responded had included children subject to immigration controls either in their plans or in their response to the Department of Health's new assessment frameworks (Department of Health *et al.*

2000). There is much talk about the care of children, the prevention of childhood poverty and the need to tackle the social exclusion of children, yet there is an absence of concern for those children who are likely to be among the most at risk:

> All face the discontinuity of exile, depriving them of familiar communities, carers and cultural backdrop against which they can develop and make the transition from childhood to adulthood. Many will not speak English as a first language. Many will be separated from their primary carer. Many will have faced traumatic events and situations in their own countries or during their journey here, including bereavement or torture. Many will be overwhelmed by their experiences in their own or in this country. Yet all the evidence demonstrates that these children receive less, not more, protection; less not more promotion of their welfare.
>
> (Refugee Children's Consortium 2000: 1)

Although unaccompanied asylum-seeking children remain the responsibility of local social services departments, they are often treated differently from other children without carers. Adele Jones's research (1998 and Chapter 6 of this volume) revealed the consequences of conflicting provisions between children's legislation and immigration legislation, and the range of ways in which children have been abused and neglected, directly by the implementation of immigration legislation, and through the gaps opened up by the contradictions. She shows that the Children Act 1989 'does not make specific reference to children affected by immigration controls, and the duty to consider the welfare of children is neglected within immigration law' (Jones 1998: 37). It is not surprising that this group of children is invisible in the policies of Social Services Departments (SSDs). Jones found that the responses of SSDs to children subject to immigration controls were variable, and in some there was no recognition that such children might come within their remit of child protection, with social workers uninterested in supporting children with immigration difficulties. Among the factors identified as contributing to this were:

- lack of comprehensive child care policy
- lack of interest and direction from senior managers
- failings of child care legislation and regulations
- issues not addressed within social work education and training
- influence of negative media, resulting in immigration cases being seen as 'undeserving'

- shifts within social work from prevention and support to crisis work and resource-led responses
- immigration not regarded as an important social work issue
- marginalisation of issues which affect black and minority ethnic families
- social work not geared to the needs of a multiracial society.

(Jones 1998: 38)

These findings are supported by the Barnardo's (2000) research, by Mynott and Humphries (2001) and by the report of the Audit Commission (2000). The Commission found that although the legal rights of unaccompanied asylum seeking children in the care of local authorities were identical to those of indigenous children, they did not receive the same standard of care, and frequently did not receive a full needs assessment or have individual care plans in place.

Jones's study found a range of ways in which social services departments were failing in their duty to children looked after by the local authority. Neglecting to identify and deal with statelessness at an early stage for example, could lead to children becoming 'overstayers' with serious consequences for young people leaving care, and seeking employment, education and housing. The requirement to appoint an 'independent visitor'[1] and to meet a child's racial, religious, linguistic and cultural needs, were found by the study to be often neglected.

Paradoxically, the issue is not only one of simple exclusion from services or neglect to carry out duties laid down by legislation. The emphasis in social work on 'protection' in child care, described above, may result in intervention at the 'heavy end' of social services powers. There is some evidence of steps having been taken to mobilise these powers against refugees and asylum seekers. For example, an attempt by council officials was made to initiate child protection proceedings against asylum seekers in the London Borough of Westminster, involving both social workers and the police. Social workers in the Borough saw this as a tactic to scapegoat the asylum seekers and refused to cooperate with the operation.[2] On this occasion the social workers and their union were not politically naïve regarding the motivation, which they saw as 'a racist operation designed to heighten ethnic tension'. This may not be the response elsewhere. Social workers are no less informed by stereotypical images of asylum seekers than other citizens. One can envisage that this combined with an obsession with 'watching their back' could lead to inappropriate, oppressive and racist intervention.

There is also evidence that children are detained under immigration act powers, even though the government's White Paper 'Fairer, Faster, Firmer' (UK Government 1998) declared that detention of a child interferes with the right to freedom, a normal life and education, and should only be used in exceptional circumstances. As Jones (1998) has shown, there is very little evidence that social workers are acting as advocates on behalf of both those children excluded from a range of benefits and from protection under the law, or indeed have an awareness of their own obligation to care for such children. A culture of ignorance and disbelief has been created where there needs to be a human rights culture.

Creeping internalisation of immigration controls

The discussion above suggests that the law and the duties of local authorities towards those in need is systematically interpreted in restrictive ways, and although this is on the face of it misplaced, it does not take place in isolation from the ways social work is being engaged in a more general disciplinary role. It is important in considering the role of social workers in immigration controls, to set the discussion in the wider context of internal controls. With regard to immigration controls, Anne Owers identifies two major ways of enforcing them:

> The first is to require the carrying of personal identification which can distinguish those legally present from those illegally on the territory. . . . The second is to spread the responsibility for enforcement among a variety of other agencies, both state and private, whose primary concern is not immigration: for example employers, benefit and housing agencies and schools.
>
> (Owers 1994: 266)

Owers makes the point that both systems are currently in operation in Britain. Although there is as yet no obligation to carry identity cards, it is common for members of visible minority communities to be stopped, usually on the pretext of a check for a criminal or traffic offence, and asked for evidence of legal residence. It is estimated that black people are six times more likely to be stopped and searched than are white people (Sivanandan 2000). And a network already exists of 'devolved immigration controllers' (Owers 1994: 267) – from teachers trying to decide which children in a class can travel on a group British passport, to housing officials, benefits officers and education and health administrators (Cohen *et al.* 1997; Hayes 2000). As the research by Cohen *et al.* confirmed, this system's operation is inconsistent and unregulated, but it is increasingly visible, with in some cases, records kept on a database that can be accessed centrally.

One does not need to be a clairvoyant to predict that the call for identity cards will be heard again soon, showing not only a photograph of the holder, but also possibly incorporating a fingerprint (see Owers 1994). In such circumstances, which groups are the most likely to come under suspicion, and to be asked to prove their 'legality'? They are of course likely to be those who are members of visible minority communities. And inevitably such a system will have limited effectiveness, and will create widespread hostility and resentment. And to the enforcement and surveillance role of social workers and other 'helping' professions, already confirmed by a raft of new legislation, will be added this formal recognition of internal policing of immigration status.

This examination of what social workers are expected to do in relation to people suffering as a result of their immigration status is illustrative of the changing role of social work in the twenty-first century. The questions facing social work, as with other welfare and health professionals, should not be concerned with how the job imposed on them can be carried out more efficiently. The questions that should concern them are with issues of ethics, politics and strategies of resistance.

Notes

1 An independent visitor is a volunteer who acts as an adult friend to children or young people looked after by a local authority, recommended by the Children Act 1989.
2 Reported in the *Socialist Worker*, 14 April 2000, 'Workers block plan to round up refugees' kids'.

References

Amnesty International, (2000) *Most vulnerable of all: the treatment of unaccompanied refugee children in the UK*, London: Amnesty International UK.
Audit Commission (2000) *Another Country: implementing dispersal under the Immigration and Asylum Act 1999*, London: Audit Commission.
Bailey, R. and Brake, M. (eds) (1975) *Radical Social Work*, London: Edward Arnold.
Barnardo's, (2000) *Children First and Foremost: meeting the needs of unaccompanied asylum-seeking children*, London: Barnardo's.
Cohen, S. (1996) 'Anti-semitism, immigration controls and the welfare state', in D. Taylor (ed.) *Critical Social Policy: a reader*, London: Sage, pp 27–47.

Cohen, S., Hayes, D., Humphries, B. and Sime, C. (1997) *Immigration Controls and Health*: *implementation of the NHS (Charges to Overseas Visitors) Regulations 1989*, Manchester: GMIAU and Manchester Metropolitan University.

Court of Appeal (Civil Division) (2000) *Case Nos*: *C/1999/0747, C/1999/7342, C/1999/7696, Judgment as approved by the Court*, Royal Courts of Justice, Thursday 22 June 2000.

Department of Health (1988) *Protecting Children*: *a guide for social workers undertaking a comprehensive assessment*, London: HMSO.

—— (1991) *Working Together under the Children Act*, London: HMSO.

—— (1998) *Quality Protects*: *framework for action and objectives for social services for children*, London: HMSO.

Department of Health, Department for Education and Employment, Home Office (2000) *Framework for the Assessment of Children in Need and their Families*, The Stationery Office, Norwich.

Duvell, F. and Jordan, B. (2000) *"How low can you go?' Dilemmas of social work with asylum seekers in London'*, Exeter: Department of Social Work, Exeter University.

Harding, J. (2000) *The Uninvited*: *refugees at the rich man's gate*, London: Routledge.

Hayes, D. (2000) 'Outsiders within: the role of welfare in the internal control of immigration', in J. Batsleer and B. Humphries (eds), *Welfare, Exclusion and Political Agency*, London: Routledge, pp 63–78.

Howe, D. (1996) 'Regulation for radicals: the state, CCETSW and the academy', in N. Parton (ed.) *Social Theory, Social Change and Social Work*, London: Routledge, pp 172–189.

Hudson, D. (1997) 'Excluded at home, excluded in the UK', *Adults Learning*, 8(5), pp 121–123.

Humphries, B. (1997) 'The dismantling of anti-discrimination in British social work: a view from social work education', *International Social Work*, 40(3): 289–301.

Jones, A. (1998) *The Child Welfare Implications of UK Immigration and Asylum Policy*, Manchester: Manchester Metropolitan University.

Jones, C. (1983) *State Social Work and the Working Class*, London: Macmillan.

—— (1993) 'Distortion and demonisation: the Right and anti-racist social work education', *Social Work Education*, 12(12): 9–16.

Jones, C. and Novak, T. (1999) *Poverty, Welfare and the Disciplinary State*, London: Routledge.

Jordan, B. (2000) *Social Work and the Third Way*: *tough love as social policy*, London: Sage.

Mynott, E. (1999) *Immigration, Asylum and the Provision of Services in Manchester*: *a preliminary report*. Manchester, Manchester Metropolitan University.

Mynott, E. and Humphries, B. (2001) *Living Your Life Across Bounderies*: *Young Separated Refugees in Greater Manchester*, London: Save the Children Fund.

Otway, O. (1996) 'Social work with children and their families: from child welfare to child protection', in N. Parton (ed.) *Social Theory, Social Change and Social Work*, London: Routledge, pp 152–171.

Owers, A.(1994) 'The age of internal controls', in S. Spencer (ed.) *Strangers and Citizens: a positive approach to migrants and refugees*, London: Rivers Oram Press, pp 264–281.

Parton, N. (1996a) 'Social theory, social change and social work: introduction', in N. Parton (ed.) *Social Theory, Social Change and Social Work*, London: Routledge, pp 4–18.

—— (ed.) (1996b) *Social Theory, Social Change and Social Work*, London: Routledge.

Rayner, J. (2001) 'Mad remedies', *The Observer*, 7 January 2001: 27.

Refugee Children's Consortium (2000) *Children First: the asylum debate and young people*, Briefing for the Labour Party Conference from the Refugee Children's Consortium.

Sivanandan, A. (2000) 'Reclaiming the struggle', *Race and Class*, 42(2): 67–73.

Social Services Inspectorate (1993) *Evaluating Performance in Child Protection: a framework for the inspection of local authority social services practice and systems*, London: HMSO.

Taylor, D. (ed.) (1996) *Critical Social Policy: a reader*, London: Sage.

UK Government (1998) *Fairer, Faster, Firmer: a modern approach to immigration and asylum*, CM4018, July, London: Stationery Office.

9   Dining with the devil

The 1999 Immigration and Asylum Act and the voluntary sector

Steve Cohen

Introduction

The 1999 Immigration and Asylum Act has been met with universal opposition from those who support the rights of asylum seekers. This opposition is understandable. The legislation represents a qualitative increase in the mistreatment, not just of refugees, but of all those subject to controls. However, there is one completely novel aspect of the 1999 Act and its implementation which appears to have attracted nil criticism, but which represents a huge reactionary development in immigration control enforcement. This is the engagement of parts of the voluntary sector in a system which is directly antagonistic to the interests of refugees. In particular it is the involvement of some voluntary agencies in that part of the legislation which transforms asylum seekers into an 'underclass' by removing entitlement to welfare state support and enforcing dependency on a new poor law. The voluntary sector, or part of it, is a designated poor law enforcer.

There are two mutually exclusive positions that can be taken on this involvement. On the one hand it can be argued that the role of the voluntary sector is essentially a facilitating one that is helpful to asylum seekers through the provision of advice and other help, based on the so-called support provisions of the 1999 Act. Linked to this is the argument that if the voluntary sector did not contract for this service then it would probably be undertaken by far more problematic organisations – such as private security companies. On the other hand it can be argued that any identification with any part of the 1999 legislation serves to legitimise and therefore strengthen not only the new poor law, but the whole of the legislation. This is the position taken by this chapter.

The role of the voluntary sector, or at least its advice-giving component, has historically been to act as an advocate against state authority. Now there is a situation where the sector has become a junior partner of the state. It is not clear how many, if any, asylum seekers have been consulted on the ethics of such a partnership. What is clear is that those voluntary sector agencies undertaking functions relating to the new legislation are receiving large amounts of government monies for this.[1] There is no reason to doubt the honourable if mistaken nature of these agencies' motives and the sincerity of the belief that they are assisting asylum seekers. However, the objective reality is that these organisations now have a financial stake in the implementation of the 1999 Act. As Virgil wrote about the Trojan horse, 'Beware the Greeks bearing gifts'. In any event it is arguable that this money would be better spent by the restoration of benefit and housing rights to asylum seekers, rights which were abolished by the Act. This chapter is not being written to condemn, but to open up discussion on the role of the voluntary sector with respect to the new legislation.

Chutzpah *and the voluntary sector's new found friend*

All those working in the voluntary sector in the UK will be acutely aware of the massive cutbacks it has suffered over the last decade. This has often happened at local level through Labour-controlled councils. The main targets have frequently been immigration advisory units. For instance, in the early 1990s Manchester City Council cut its grant to both the Greater Manchester Immigration Aid Unit and South Manchester Law Centre. More recently Liverpool has completely closed down the Merseyside Immigration Aid Unit and Birmingham has pulled the plug on the Independent Immigration Advisory Service. These attacks have often been linked to accusations that voluntary sector agencies are 'too political' or are not providing 'value for money'.

This antagonism towards the voluntary sector ought itself to be a warning against the Home Office's fulsome praise for that sector as a potential ally in the implementation of the 1999 legislation. This newfound admiration is seen in the White Paper *Fairer, Faster and Firmer: a modern approach to immigration and asylum* (Home Office 1998), precursor to the legislation. This stated that 'the Government is particularly concerned to explore ways of harnessing the energy and expertise of voluntary and independent sector bodies in providing support for asylum seekers' (para. 8.23).

What is meant by 'energy and expertise' is spelt out in far greater detail in another Home Office document – *Asylum Seekers' Support* (Home Office 1999), produced by the Asylum Seekers' Support Project Team of the Immigration and Nationality Directorate (IND). In a chapter headed 'Voluntary and community involvement' it contains a section on 'what the voluntary sector can offer'. What it can offer is apparently:

- *volunteers*: the voluntary sector's unique capacity to involve volunteers in their work has major benefits . . .
- *additional resources*: once voluntary agencies are involved in the support arrangements, they will start to raise funds to provide additional services . . .
- *expertise*: the expertise in meeting the support needs of asylum seekers is almost exclusively based in the voluntary sector . . .
- *networking capacity*: a great strength of the voluntary sector agencies is their ability to draw in other organisations in the sector to provide additional resources or expertise . . .
- *policy development*: the voluntary sector has a good record in developing imaginative responses . . .

These are all genuine and important attributes of the voluntary sector. Indeed they have consistently, though usually unsuccessfully, been articulated by that sector itself in attempting to defend itself against cutbacks. It is therefore quite understandable to be suspicious of a government using these very same arguments in justifying voluntary sector involvement in a highly repressive piece of legislation. It is worthy of even more suspicion in that the Home Office, having witnessed cutbacks to the voluntary sector, now expects that same sector to accumulate 'additional resources' to help asylum seekers in respect to whom the government is now depriving of welfare state support. There is a Yiddish word for this – *chutzpah*.[2]

The repressive nature of the 1999 Act

The 1999 Act does not exist in historic isolation. It is simply the latest piece in a long line of immigration control legislation going back to the 1905 Aliens Act. Even within the last decade, it was preceded by the 1993 Asylum and Immigration Appeals Act, and the 1996 Asylum and Immigration Act. In this context the 1999 Act is just another brick in the wall. Apart from anything else this shows the futility of demanding the repeal at any given time of the latest piece of legislation – as the rest of the wall remains. However, the 1999 Act does represent what is probably the greatest tightening of controls since 1905. It is a leap from quantity into quality. It is against this background that the involvement of the voluntary sector has to be judged, both politically and ethically.

The major changes effected by the Act include the following: first it slashes the immigration appeal system by removing any separate right of appeal against deportation. This will accelerate the whole process of removal from the UK and will as a consequence make it far harder to campaign against any particular removal. Second, it allows for a financial bond to be imposed on anyone wanting to come to the UK or on their sponsor as a guarantee they will return home. This is effectively a restriction on the poor. Third, it grants immigration officers powers to arrest, search and fingerprint – roughly equivalent to that of the police – though without any independent body to investigate abuse.

Big Brother

There is one conspicuous feature running right through the legislation. This is the elevation of the state machinery into the role of Big Brother in its surveillance of asylum seekers. Sections 18 and 19 enable the immigration service to demand information from carrying companies about passengers and the arrival of ships, aircraft or trains carrying non-European Economic Association (EEA) citizens.[3] The Act obliges existing policing agencies to pass on immigration control information to the Home Office. Section 20 provides for information to be supplied 'for immigration purposes' to the Home Secretary by the police, the National Criminal Intelligence Service, the National Crime Squad and HM Customs and Excise. Section 20 also allows the Home Secretary to make an order obliging a 'specified person' to pass on information for 'immigration purposes'. The danger is that such specified persons may be anyone working within the voluntary sector. Section 24 obliges registrars to report to the Home Office marriages considered to be 'sham' – an obligation that simply regularises much of present practice. Section 127 obliges the postal service to provide information about any request from an asylum seeker for the redirection of post.

The Asylum Support Regulations 2000, drawn up under the Act, oblige supported asylum seekers to disclose an unprecedented amount of personal information (Regulation 15). Under the regulations an asylum seeker must inform the Home Office's National Asylum Support Service (NASS) immediately and in writing if she or he: (a) is joined in the United Kingdom by a dependant; (b) receives or gains access to any money; (c) becomes employed; (d) becomes unemployed; (e) changes his or her name; (f) gets married; (g) starts living with a person as if married to that person; (h) gets divorced; (i) separates from a spouse, or from a person with whom he or she has been living as if married to that person; (j) becomes pregnant; (k) has a child; (l) leaves school; (m) starts to share accommodation with another person; (n) moves to a different address; (o) goes into hospital; (p) goes to prison or is otherwise held in custody; (q) leaves the United Kingdom; (r) dies.

Exclusion from welfare state support

The role assigned to the voluntary sector in the enforcement of the 1999 Act is directly related to Part VI of the Act. Part VI is inappropriately entitled 'support for asylum seekers'. It is inappropriate because what this Part does is to exclude from means-tested and non-contributory benefits all persons subject to immigration control. In addition, local authority housing, both homelessness accommodation and allocation from the housing register, are likewise to be denied to those subject to immigration control. The definition of people 'subject to immigration control' is far wider than asylum seekers. In particular, it includes all those whose leave to enter or remain in the UK is subject to a condition that they do not have recourse to public funds. This embraces the vast majority of those non-British or non-EEA nationals entering the UK, for instance visitors, students and those allowed in for family settlement such as spouses, young children or elderly parents.

The effect of Part VI is to sever the link between migrants, immigrants and refugees with entitlement to primary welfare state provision on the level of the national or local state. This has been a long-term historic development stretching back to the origins of welfare at the start of the twentieth century (Cohen 1996). It was given a major boost by the 1993 and 1996 legislation. Following the 1996 Act, immigration lawyers established significant legal precedents, imposing obligations on local authorities to support asylum seekers and others under the 1948 National Assistance Act (Section 21) and the 1989 Children Act (Section 17). Predictably, the 1999 Act abolished these legislative avenues of support for those subject to controls.

The new poor law safety net

Part VI substitutes welfare state provision for asylum seekers with a so-called support scheme. The essential components of this are as follows. First, the new scheme is a national one administered by the newly created National Asylum Support Service (NASS). This body is hardly impartial. It is part of the Immigration and Nationality Directorate (IND) of the Home Office. Its Director adopts government rhetoric as to the purpose of the new scheme – namely, 'to discourage those who apply for asylum on economic grounds' (Zetter and Pearl 1999:

Foreword). A NASS pamphlet *The New Asylum Support Scheme* issued in March 2000, is quite clear that NASS is not neutral when it comes to the expulsion of failed asylum seekers and particularly the expulsion of failed asylum-seeking families with children (the latter being entitled to support after refusal of the asylum claim up to the date of expulsion). The pamphlet states 'It is, therefore, important that we develop our removals capacity to ensure that we can effectively remove such families from the country' (para. 8.32). Second, the scheme excludes asylum seekers from the money economy and places them in a feudal cashless economy. It achieves this through providing not money but vouchers to asylum seekers. Except in the case of refugees under eighteen years old, these vouchers are valued at just 70 per cent of income support level. They are only redeemable at those shops that have agreed to enter the scheme. Shops are not obliged to provide change in cash or any other form where vouchers are under-spent. Third, accommodation is to be provided under the scheme via contracts entered into with NASS by local authorities, private landlords or housing associations (now known as registered social landlords, RSLs). As is seen below this provision of accommodation is central to the involuntary/compulsory dispersal of asylum seekers.

Role given to the voluntary sector

The significance given by the Home Office to the voluntary sector in implementing the support provisions of the 1999 Act can be seen in the constant references in Home Office documentation to the need for voluntary agency involvement. Examples have been given above in respect to the documents *Fairer, Faster and Firmer* (Home Office 1998) and *Asylum Seekers' Support* (Home Office 1999). NASS provides constant positive affirmation of voluntary sector involvement. For instance, a letter of 4 February 2000 from the Director of NASS to its 'stakeholder' group says 'I am pleased to say that we are making very good progress with the voluntary sector who are essentially providing two key elements of the scheme: reception assistants and one-stop services'.

One-stop services are described in the NASS pamphlet *The New Asylum Support Scheme* as 'services (which) will be the focal point for harnessing voluntary and community support throughout the region to assist asylum seekers' (para. 9). These services will also be of an advice nature, such as advising on local facilities and legal representation. In practice, reception assistants operate as part of the one-stop services.

It is the role of reception assistants which is particularly indicative of the huge compromises expected of the voluntary sector. This role is spelt out in the *Draft Process Manual for the Asylum Support System* (Home Office 1999, Chapter 2).[4] Two main functions are helping claimants complete an application form for assistance from NASS and the provision of emergency accommodation and support whilst NASS considers the application. Under the grant agreement with NASS agencies can place asylum seekers in emergency accommodation for only seven days whilst a decision is made on their eligibility for support. If support is refused then the grant agreements cease funding of emergency accommodation, even where the refusal is being appealed. This places voluntary agencies in a position of colluding in the eviction of asylum seekers. A letter of 3 November 2000 from the Policy Unit at NASS[5] explains that reception assistants also have the role of providing emergency support of meals and other 'essential living needs', and that this means ceasing to provide such support once NASS has determined eligibility. So where NASS refuses even voucher help, then the voluntary agency is in effect being asked to condemn asylum seekers to starvation as well as homelessness. The *Process Manual* is very clear about this and about the way that the voluntary sector is to be NASS's puppet in starving out asylum seekers. The manual says, in respect of these emergency needs pending a decision on eligibility, the objective of the Immigration and Nationality Directorate is 'to provide resources for the voluntary sector to provide safety net support to those who appear to be destitute . . . to maintain control of provision so that as soon as a rejection decision is made, support is withdrawn' (para. 2.30).

The functions of reception assistants can be understood only in relation to another highly dubious role, namely that of trying to persuade asylum seekers not to make a claim on NASS in the first place. The *Process Manual* states that a policy objective of the reception assistant scheme is that 'appropriate and timely advice is given to asylum seekers to enable them to identify alternatives to Directorate support and to take up offers of support outside the safety net scheme' (para. 2.5). What this means is that asylum seekers should be 'open to encouragement to seek support from friends and family and be assisted in contacting friends, family or others in their communities who may be able to support and/or accommodate them. They will be expected to show within reason that they have exhausted all avenues of approach to contacts even where this is not their preferred option' (para. 2.1).

In other words, voluntary sector agencies, whose role is normally to assist claimants in accessing and maximising state benefits, are now expected to actively discourage asylum seekers from applying for even the poor law support left to them.

And assumed by the voluntary sector

Participating agencies have not had these roles thrust upon them. They have readily assumed them. This is clear from a February 1999 document, *The Role and Funding of the Voluntary Sector in Relation to the Proposed Asylum Support Process*, produced by the so-called Asylum Support Voluntary Action Group. This included the main voluntary sector refugee agencies: the Refugee Council, Refugee Action and the Refugee Arrivals Project. However the Group was established by the Home Office and included representatives from the IND, hardly a guarantee that the interests of asylum seekers were paramount. The document strongly endorsed voluntary sector involvement in the support scheme. Again, the endorsement is inevitably politically suspect, given Home Office collaboration. For instance the document itemises the 'strengths' of the voluntary sector (para. 3.2.2) – an itemisation that was subsequently reproduced in the document *Asylum Seekers' Support* discussed above. Again the voluntary sector's use of volunteers was perceived as a 'strength'. However it is made clear that this strength derives from the unpaid nature of volunteers' work. It states 'volunteers, simply by the work that they do, increase the capacity of organisations and enable agencies to carry out tasks that they would otherwise not have the funds to do'. This cost-cutting exercise is hardly in the interests of asylum seekers let alone those of the volunteers. It's another example of *chutzpah.*

There is some ambiguous recognition in the document that there may be a 'perceived potential conflict of interest' within the role being assumed by the voluntary sector. This recognition is neither clearly articulated nor resolved. The document states: 'It may be suggested that there might be a conflict of interests between the objectives and policies of the asylum support system and what voluntary agencies perceive to be the interests of their clients, and that the involvement of voluntary agencies might therefore undermine the support system'(para. 3.2.3). The perceived conflict is not spelt out. Ultimately, though this seems deliberately unstated, it can only be based on the dichotomy between a voluntary sector role in helping asylum seekers and the Home Office's role in removing them. This dichotomy seems to boil down within the document to a concern that it 'might be argued that the voluntary sector would not be sufficiently rigorous in exploring alternative options' (para. 4.4.3). In other words there is a concern that the reception assistants will not encourage claimants to seek support outside of the NASS support system, thereby saving the Home Office from providing even poor law support. In practice, this concern is about the voluntary sector 'taking sides' on behalf of asylum seekers. This writer is fully in favour of this happening. However the document, which is in the name of major voluntary sector agencies, is quick to reassure it will not happen. It states, in respect to fears that the agencies will not direct claimants away from the NASS scheme, 'we do not accept this view. All the specialist refugee voluntary agencies and projects have a good track record of working objectively within the funding criteria they have been given' (para. 3.2.3). It later says 'Furthermore, the basis on which support and accommodation are offered will simply not make it an attractive option to asylum seekers who have other possibilities open to them. Finally a process of the monitoring of referrals will enable problems to be identified at an early stage and corrective action taken' (para. 4.4.3). The voluntary sector organisations which gave their names to this document are quite willing that the Home Office police their role and take 'corrective action' against them if they fall out of line. This is just the opposite of that sector's historic function of acting as an advocate on behalf of clients against state authority.

The NASS letter of 3 November 2000 refers to further voluntary sector engagement with NASS. There exists a 'stakeholder group', which meets 'as and when necessary to provide support and consultation on issues relevant to NASS'. The voluntary agencies in the group include National Associations of Citizens Advice Bureaux, Amnesty International and the Terrance Higgins Trust. Not only do representatives from NASS attend the meetings but so also do those from the Integrated Casework Directorate of the Immigration and Nationality Directorate and from the Association of Chief Police Officers. Again, there seems to have been no attempt to determine the views of asylum seekers on these collusive meetings involving both the police and the section of the IND that is responsible for deciding on the fate of refugees and their asylum claims.

Other parts of the voluntary sector: refugee community organisations

Engagement by its advice-giving component is not the only involvement by the voluntary sector intended by the Home Office in the implementation of the 1999 Act. Once again, these other components have escaped criticism for an actual or potential engagement. For instance, right through the documentation there are references to refugee community organisations (RCOs) as playing an important role within the new support system. RCOs range from small bodies run on voluntary labour to some large charities with premises and significant local authority or trust income. The document on the role and funding of the voluntary sector in relation to the proposed asylum support process details a role for RCOs. This includes helping 'informally and formally with assistants in all elements of the pre-assessment process . . . providing emergency accommodation and facilitating contact with families and friends; participating in the provision of support and accommodation packages; contributing to the development of mutual understanding between refugees and the host community; providing cultural and recreational activities; providing an effective self-help mechanism for those allowed to stay' (para. 4.3.2).

On the face of it this involvement by community organisations would seem to be positive and enhancing. However there is an alternative and politically more realistic way of viewing this issue. This is that it is wrong for the state to offload its obligations towards asylum seekers onto refugee communities through individuals or organisations. This creates a form of collective responsibility. It is redolent of the (mis)treatment by the British government of the Jewish community and Jewish asylum seekers from Nazism in the 1930s. Only a small minority of Jews was given permission to enter the UK. The majority of these only managed to enter because members of the leadership of the Jewish community at a meeting with the Home Secretary on 7 April 1933, agreed that no refugee would become 'a charge on public funds' and the various Jewish refugee committees undertook to support refugees financially (Sherman 1973: 30). So today it is equally intolerable that often financially impoverished refugee communities, are being expected to support 'their own'.

Registered social landlords

Housing Associations (now known as registered social landlords, RSLs), are another component of the voluntary sector which has uncritically assumed a role in administering the 1999 legislation. RSLs have signed contracts with NASS to provide housing to asylum seekers pending a decision on the substantive asylum claim. This is being actively encouraged by the Housing Corporation[6] which has produced lengthy Guidelines for RSLs (Zetter and Pearl 1999). It is undoubtedly the case that many RSLs have over the years provided a very positive service to refugees. Examples are 'Mosscare' in Manchester and 'St Mungo's' in Lambeth. However, by contracting with NASS and thus helping implement the 1999 Act, RSLs are giving credibility to a pernicious housing system which again bears every resemblance to the poor laws.

Examples of this perniciousness are as follows. First, asylum seekers are given no choice as to the locality in which they are housed. In this very real sense the whole scheme is predicated on forced dispersal. The government stated in its White Paper *Fairer, Faster and Firmer* that 'asylum seekers would be expected to take what was available, and would not be able to pick and choose where they were accommodated' (Home Office 1998: para. 8.22). Second, occupants accommodated under the scheme are deprived of protection against eviction under the 1977 Evictions Act. Landlords do not have to go through the courts to effect eviction. Third, the Housing Corporation is urging that possibly inferior accommodation be provided to asylum seekers. Housing Corporation Circular R3–23/99 states 'RSLs in cluster areas may, in consultation with the local authority, use existing hard to let stock . . . to house asylum seekers' (Zetter and Pearl 1999: 37)

Fourth, the housing scheme is regarded by the Home Office as a further method of surveillance, and of further exercising its Big Brother function over asylum seekers. The whole scheme is a snoopers' charter. Some examples are contained within the 1999 Act itself. Section 100 obliges local authorities or RSLs to disclose to the Home Secretary whatever information about housing accommodation is requested. Section 126 obliges the owner or manager of property accommodating asylum seekers under the Act to supply information about the occupants. Other examples of this surveillance are contained in the Asylum Support Regulations 2000 drawn up under the 1999 Act. Asylum seekers are to be tied to accommodation as the Victorian poor were tied to the workhouse. The Support Regulations say asylum seekers and dependants cannot be absent for more than seven consecutive days and nights or more than a total of fourteen days and nights in any six-month period, without the permission of the Home Office (Regulation 20) – which presumably means NASS. Breach of this requirement can lead to eviction.

Finally if an asylum seeker is refused refugee status and has exhausted all immigration appeals then NASS will cease financial support and any contract with a housing provider terminates. The Housing Corporation Guidelines say, 'this arrangement is one which RSLs will be required to manage in a sensitive but efficient manner' (Zetter and Pearl 1999: 46). In practice most RSLs will simply not be able to afford to allow failed asylum seekers to remain rent-free and will move to eviction. The Guidelines state that 'RSLs should develop a policy which provides clear guidelines about the determination of contracts and provide adequate training for how staff should execute such actions'. This is just a euphemistic way of saying RSL staff must be prepared to put asylum seekers onto the streets. More than any other factor, this illustrates why it is politically and ethically untenable for the voluntary sector, however laudable its motives, to be involved in the implementation of what is essentially anti-refugee legislation.

The politics of accepting Home Office monies

There is nothing necessarily wrong in principle for the voluntary sector to accept government monies for projects, though it does require constant political vigilance to ensure that the source of funding does not constrain its use. It is a matter of balancing needs with risks. However, there does come a point where the risks are so obviously huge that accepting monies becomes highly questionable. The most obvious example of this is the acceptance of Home Office funds to challenge the Home Office on the issue of asylum and immigration control. The contradiction is just too great. Moreover, any and all professional involvement with immigration controls ought to be premised on the basis of challenging these controls and not passively accepting them. This is because the whole immigration control enterprise is antagonistic to the interests of migrants, immigrants and refugees.

Even prior to the 1999 Act the Home Office was providing funding to some voluntary sector agencies in respect of controls. But this is tainted money. For example the Immigration Advisory Service and the Refugee Legal Centre were established by the Government, and are mainly funded by the Home Office to offer legal advice and representation. Both agencies do some excellent work. However neither, because of their funding source, have the freedom to mount campaigns seriously challenging controls. This can be contrasted with the Medical Foundation for the Care of Victims of Torture, a unique venture helping refugees subjected to torture to gain asylum. In her evidence to the House of Commons Special Standing Committee on the Immigration and Asylum Bill (18 March 1999), a representative from the Foundation emphasised that it took no Home Office monies as a sign of its independence.

So what should the voluntary sector be doing?

The 1999 Act is not to be condemned because it institutes a national scheme for asylum seekers. All else being equal, any civilised response to the plight of asylum seekers demands a national scheme drawing on the support of a whole range of agencies, including voluntary sector agencies. The reason the Act is to be absolutely condemned is because it creates a situation where nothing is equal.

The involvement of some voluntary sector agencies in implementing the 1999 legislation can be understood as part of a wider process whereby immigration control enforcement is no longer the preserve of the immigration or police service. It now encompasses both large areas of local government and of the private sector. It encompasses local government through its responsibilities for administering benefits (such as housing and council tax benefits) and services (such as higher education and housing), which are linked to immigration status. The 1999 legislation adds significant areas of community care to local authority services tied to immigration status.[7] What all this means is that local authority workers are required to investigate immigration status.

Ever since the 1996 Asylum and Immigration Act, employers (including private employers) have become criminally liable for employing workers ineligible to work because of their immigration status. This ensures that employers are now directly concerned in immigration control enforcement. As a result of the 1987 Immigration (Carriers Liability) Act (now replaced and extended by Part 2 of the 1999 Act), carrying companies are brought into the sphere of immigration control enforcement by the penalising of carriers for transporting hidden or incorrectly documented passengers.

The only responsible position that can be taken by voluntary agencies is one of non-cooperation with the 1999 legislation, linked to a campaign for the reinstatement of welfare state provision for asylum seekers. Helping implement the legislation in itself undermines any campaign against it.

Examples of non-cooperation

This call for non-cooperation is not political purism. There are already instances where the major voluntary sector refugee organisations have not complied with everything demanded by the Home Office and this non-compliance represents hope for future good practice. In particular, they have refused to administer the Dickensian 'hard cases' fund established by NASS outside of the statutory framework to supposedly support some asylum seekers after a refusal of their asylum claim (after which time statutory support ceases, except in the case of children, or families with children).[8] This 'hard cases' fund is essentially charity, which NASS can distribute or withhold from whomever it wants. Asylum seekers should be entitled to rights and not have to beg for charity. It is quite correct for voluntary sector agencies to refuse to have anything to do with the fund.

On 31 October 2000, Refugee Action circulated a letter saying it had closed down its Liverpool office offering one-stop and reception services. Though this withdrawal was not presented as one of principle, for instance Refugee Action kept open its Manchester office, yet its criticisms were devastating and went to the core of the scheme. The circulated letter stated that:

> Asylum seekers' unmet needs for basic safety, comfort and maintenance are so acute, so widespread and so fundamental that they are beyond the resources of the voluntary sector to provide. . . . Many have not received the vouchers they need in order to buy food. . . . Many do not receive travel vouchers enabling them to attend their all-important asylum interviews with the Immigration Service. Many feel desperately unsafe or insecure in sub-standard accommodation. . . . NASS decision-making is unacceptably slow and monitoring of local accommodation standards has been poor. . . . The result is an unacceptably high level of racial harassment and attack. Last week a 4-year-old child was hospitalised with suspected concussion. He had been hit by a brick, thrown through the window of his home.

The Guardian reported one positive example within the retail trade of voluntary sector non-cooperation (3 April and 15 April 2000). The charities Oxfam, Barnardo's, Shelter, Marie Curie Foundation and Save the Children Fund have refused to accept the new vouchers in their shops – at least in their present form where change cannot be given. Oxfam, which has 840 charity shops, has called upon major retailers to follow its example.

For total defiance

These examples, though limited in number, are in reality examples of defiance. They establish a principle and the principle is one of non-cooperation by the voluntary sector with aspects of the new poor law. What I am arguing is that this principle be extended so as to cover the entirety of the poor law established by the so-called support provisions of the 1999 Immigration and Asylum Act. This withdrawal of co-operation would, especially if linked to community protest, encourage other participating bodies, in particular local authorities, to do the same. Such powerful action could force the Home Office into restoring all welfare state entitlements to asylum seekers.

Integration or anti-racism?

Non-cooperation by the voluntary sector with the state machinery should encompass the entirety of immigration control. There are no benevolent or progressive aspects of control. There is just one inter-locked racist and reactionary system. This has become of renewed relevance with the publication of *Full and Equal Citizens: a strategy for the integration of refugees into the United Kingdom* (Home Office 2000). This has a section on the voluntary sector role. The whole document, and the project behind it, is extremely problematic. It is based on nation-alistic and chauvinistic notions of acculturisation – of refugees being only truly acceptable once truly assimilated. So refugees are to be offered 'orientation courses' which 'would provide information on British citizenship and increase awareness and understanding of how the main institutions and authorities in the UK work' (Home Office 2000: 6). However the most objectionable facet of this whole project is that it is explicitly exclusive. It is to be orchestrated by a National Refugee Integration Forum, and this Forum is to be chaired by NASS. Given the central role of NASS it is not surprising that much assistance available under the scheme is to be denied to asylum seekers, and is to be provided only to that small minority granted recognised refugee status or excep-tional leave to remain. In other words the whole 'integration' project is constructed on the implementation of the grossly restrictionist 1999 leg-islation. As such it would be better described as a 'disintegration' project and ought to be rejected in total by the voluntary sector.

Notes

1 According to a Refugee Action document, *Asylum Advice Teams*, sent out in January 2000 to job applicants, the Home Office had agreed to give £8 million annually for a period of two years collectively to Refugee Action, The Refugee Council, Refugee Arrivals Project, Migrant Helpline and the Scottish Refugee Council. This was to 'provide reception assistance to help new asylum applicants into the new support system under the Act; organize emergency accommodation for new applicants; provide advice and infor-mation and referral to other sources of help for asylum seekers newly dispersed to Home Office contracted accommodation (sometimes called "One Stop shops"); and give advice to successful or unsuccessful appli-cants on leaving the Home Office system'.

2 Unmitigated *cheek*. Leo Rosten defines it as 'that quality enshrined in a man who, having killed his mother and father, throws himself on the mercy of the court because he is an orphan'. For more on *chutzpah* and other Yiddish words in English, see Rosten, L. (1971) *The Joys of Yiddish*, London: Penguin.

3 The EEA comprises all European Union countries plus Iceland, Liechtenstein and Norway.

4 This manual has now been replaced by the NASS *Caseworker Instruction Manual*, a definitive version of which is not available at the time of writing. Information on its contents can be provided 'subject to costs incurred which may be charged . . . under paragraph 7 of the Code of Practice on Access. . . . In such cases the work may be charged for on the basis of an hourly rate of £20 to cover costs'. So much for freedom of information! It isn't even free.

5 Personal correspondence with the author.

6 The Housing Corporation is a UK government agency providing social housing in England.

7 For instance, Section 45 of the Health Services and Public Health Act 1968 (promotion by local authorities of the welfare of old people), and Section 12 of the Social Work (Scotland) Act 1968 (general social welfare services of Scottish local authorities).

8 In a letter of 4 April 2000 from the Refugees Integration Section at NASS to the Refugees Arrival Project at Heathrow airport, it was said that the criterion for eligibility for 'Hard Cases' support, is whether it is impracticable to travel back to the country of origin, 'by reason of physical impediment', or 'the circumstances of the case are exceptional'. 'Hard Cases' support consists of 'basic full accommodation outside London. The ex-asylum seeker will have no access to other vouchers or cash. The ex-asylum seekers must also subject themselves to regular monthly reviews in which they will be expected to demonstrate the steps they have taken to enable themselves to leave the country. If there is not sufficient evidence that this has happened then hard cases support will be terminated'.

References

Cohen, S. (1996) 'Anti-Semitism, immigration control and the welfare state', in D. Taylor (ed.) *Critical Social Policy: a reader*, London: Sage.

Home Office (1998) *Fairer, Faster, Firmer: a modern approach to immigration and asylum*, London: HMSO.

—— (1999) *Asylum Seekers' Support*, London: HMSO.

—— (2000) *Full and Equal Citizens: a strategy for the integration of refugees into the United Kingdom*, London: HMSO.

Sherman, A.J. (1973) *Island Refuge*, Paul Elek.

Zetter, R. and Pearl, M. (1999) *Guidelines for registered social landlords on the provision of housing and support services for asylum seekers*, London: Housing Corporation.

10   From safety net to exclusion

Ending social security in the UK for 'persons from abroad'

Terry Patterson

Introduction

The Conservatives' 1979 election manifesto promised 'firm action' against 'illegal immigrants' and an inquiry into the creation of a system of internal immigration controls (Gordon 1989: 6). The inquiry did not take place upon election, but many other intrusive actions subsequently did. By the start of the new century, with a softer-spoken New Labour Government, benefit entitlement has effectively ended for those previously classified as 'persons from abroad', and a system of controls is widespread and aggressively pursued.

In this chapter, I chart the insidious growth of forms of immigration control, residence and asylum seeker restrictions in social security provision over the last two decades in the United Kingdom. Within these chronologies of disentitlements, restrictive practices and occasional 'sweeteners' of positive measures, I consider evidence of liberal and illiberal policy-making, trajectories and racist effects, from a perspective of welfare rights advice. Advice workers operate in the 'buffer zone' across policy formulation and implementation, with varying degrees of conservative, liberal or radical intent and practice.

With consolidating European developments and greater global movements and conflicts in this latest 'age of migration', I look at how policies were justified and received. In processes which often deny human needs and fail human rights, I consider consequences for claimants, communities, advisers and staff in public provision, and the effectiveness of challenges to the changes. I examine the approaches of two recent commentaries on immigration and asylum policy to suggest some underpinnings and contexts to my assessment of social security changes and effects. In my conclusion, I will return briefly to these frameworks.

Perspectives

The way in which immigration and nationality acts and the immigration rules have been designed and administered to restrict the entry of black and Asian people is well documented (Dummett and Nichol 1990; Layton-Henry 1992; Spencer 1997). However, Hansen's (2000) study describes 'exceptional liberality' in British migration and nationality policy in the 1950s and subsequent 'restrictiveness'. He asserts that with a liberal elite and an illiberal public, current restrictive practices result not from failures of policy makers, but from a hostile electorate and institutional weaknesses, notably the absence in the period of an activist bill of rights or entrenched constitutional limits on political action. In apologist vein, he finds 'throwing accusations of racism at the government' to be almost 'entirely unhelpful'. He finds primary immigration to the UK from the Commonwealth as 'devoid of public support' and producing 'undesired outcomes', prior to the closure moves of the Commonwealth Immigration Act 1962. Overall, he concludes that:

> In the light of the anti-immigrant hysteria that reigned in the 1960s, and the consistent opposition towards immigration that has prevailed throughout the post-war period, the only remarkable element of Britain's current migration policies is that they are not more restrictive.
>
> (Hansen 2000: 244)

Geddes asserts that 'immigration policies are configured by tensions between control and expansion and between inclusion and exclusion' (Geddes 2000: 16), and he advocates an institutionalist approach in assessing how a Europeanised migration issues agenda structures prospects. Following Castles and Miller (1998), he notes the general trends of globalisation, acceleration, differentiation, feminisation and politicisation, which succinctly summarise the increasing scale of migratory movements, with familiar distinctions involving skilled labour, guest workers, family reunion and asylum seeking. Geddes also notes that in the rhetoric of restriction, 'policy failure' may harden commitments to further restrictions rather than lead to re-evaluation or acknowledgement of widespread 'implementation gaps' (Geddes 2000: 24).

Both Hansen and Geddes put domestic and European policy-making on immigration and citizenship into sharp relief. The domestic rhetoric is of 'firm but fair' policies. At European level it is characterised as 'to consolidate foreign communities which have taken on the characteristics of permanence' and to strengthen co-operation between member states in the campaign against illegal immigration and employment. Other accounts chart restrictionist legal approaches to asylum in the UK (Harvey 2000), and the racialised treatment of refugees and asylum in Britain (Shah 2000), in the context of international obligations and European developments. Approving Joppke's comments on damaging effects of the conflation of asylum and immigration, Geddes notes that:

> . . . the harsh discourse and practice of anti-immigration politics has been redirected towards the soft target of asylum seekers. . . . There is no more potent contemporary myth than the immigrant 'welfare scrounger'.
>
> (Geddes 2000: 29, 167)

There are contradictions here. The conflation of categories has been used politically to denounce asylum seekers as 'economic migrants', whereas in reality the categories are breaking down, owing to widespread unrest and poverty across the globe. Restrictionist agendas are fundamentally at odds with increased communication and transport links, with greater movements of population and with ethical redress of global poverty and exploitative regimes.

Within this wide canvas, my focus is on the UK social security dimensions, including the extent of scrutiny, fairness and support. National citizenship of an EU state is the basis for free movement rights within the EU and resultant social entitlements, whereas legal residence and contributions are now the general basis of entitlements in national welfare states. I turn first to the internal control aspects of social security in the UK, before considering new residence rules and asylum seeking.

Immigration controls, racial discrimination and social security

Social security has a history of achievements, in redressing poverty, and of failure, in maintaining destitution. Within recent decades of retrenchment, policy-making includes many episodes of the creation of moral panics. For example, these have presented young people as living in luxury at the expense of the state – facilitating cuts in 1985 for young people in board and lodging; in 1988 with withdrawal of benefits for 16–17 year olds and reduced rates for under-25-year-olds; and in 1996 with the introduction of a low 'single room rent' for under-25-year-olds claiming housing benefit. There has been similar scapegoating of other 'non-deserving' groups, such as single parents, with hardship in

1993 under the Child Support Act, and in 1997 when single parent benefits were abolished. These cuts have continued across Conservative and Labour governments. The treatment of people arriving from abroad gives an illuminating insight within these patterns. It has a long history, and in the 1950s for example, the Assistance Board, then administering national assistance benefits, found it necessary to be severe towards 'the feckless, the "work-shy" and the coloured immigrant' (Titmuss 1976: 227).

Scrutiny in the 1980s

The modern history of 'public funds' restrictions for people coming from abroad, and racial inequality in benefits was summarised in studies in the 1980s (Gordon and Newnham 1985, Storey 1986). These highlighted the piecemeal introduction of internal immigration measures into social security, with damaging consequences for those concerned, for civil liberties and for 'the sense of security of ethnic minorities generally' (Storey 1986: 195). They note milestones, such as the 1980 supplementary benefit rules which introduced a formal exclusion of 'persons from abroad', replacing a discretionary power to deny benefit in individual cases. These rules also created a legal power to make sponsors liable to maintain dependants. Similarly, the Divisional Court in 1981 gave 'the first clear, practical definition of public funds' (Gordon and Newnham 1985: 9).

The category of 'persons from abroad' covered people with 'limited leave' and 'no recourse to public funds' in this country under immigration rules, as well as 'overstayers', people subject to deportation orders and those with 'illegal entry' (Chapeltown CAB and Harehills and Chapeltown Law Centre 1983). Most people settled in the UK, along with other groups such as EEC nationals or people with exceptional leave, continued to be fully entitled to supplementary benefit in the normal way. People with a temporary disruption of funds from abroad, and people applying to vary leave or appealing immigration decisions could still claim weekly Urgent Needs Allowances under Urgent Cases rules.

From the start, the supplementary benefit rules were very difficult for the public, advisers and staff alike, with complications for partners, fiancé(e)s and children, and further dilemmas of when to avoid making a claim of 'public funds', even with a lawful entitlement to benefit. Claiming public funds inadvertently or in breach of immigration conditions could prejudice later decisions about permission to stay, or could lead to deportation. Support and training networks for advisers have been necessary but under-resourced. There has often been an anxiety in advice-giving, with under-confidence, frustration or swift referral to 'experts'. The 1980s accounts note widespread errors in administration of benefits, racist effects of passport checking and discouragement of legitimate claims in ethnic minority communities. Involvement of DHSS, NHS, education, housing and immigration staff, as well as the police, was sketched out. The reports note a lack of evidence of fraud or unmerited claims. Furthermore, in seeking to have racist quotes dropped from major research by the Policy Studies Institute (PSI), the DHSS 'appears to have suppressed evidence which cast some light on the racist sentiments of some staff' (Gordon and Newham 1985: 64–65). The PSI study had commented:

> Prejudices common in society at large were reflected very clearly by the staff. At one office, the researcher had only just arrived at one office when the manager jovially recounted a story about a big black buck nigger. At this office racist comments were frequent. (p. 65)

In 1985 the DHSS did publish translated *Which Benefit?* guides and planned training for staff to be aware of 'the danger and pitfalls' which occur 'when people from different cultures communicate and the skills which can assist in overcoming such problems' (Gordon and Newnham 1985: 64). At the same time, internal DHSS guidance, 'S' Circular S50/85, on the prevention of fraud, advised staff that they should be particularly careful when checking documents of a person who 'has newly arrived in the area (including people from abroad)' (Child Poverty Action Group 1986: 1).

The wider policy agenda was shaped by the 1985 'Fowler Reviews', and the resultant Social Security Act 1986. Black and minority ethnic claimants were more likely to lose out than to gain under the 'rough justice' of the package, which sought a simplification of benefits and overall cuts to aid a computerisation strategy at the DHSS. The national Committee for Non Racist Benefits (CNRB) was one oppositional group formed by advice and activist networks in 1985 to lobby against the harmful effects of the changes, and to map out anti-racist alternatives. One of its demands was that immigration control had no place in social security provision, which should be dedicated to meeting essential welfare needs in prescribed circumstances. At almost every turn of social security curtailments, groups such as the CNRB, Commission for Racial Equality, Child Poverty Action Group, National Association of Citizen's Advice Bureaux and others submitted detailed responses to government with extensive analysis and case studies of negative impacts (e.g. Social Security Committee 1996; Committee for Non Racist Benefits 1998).

The 1988 Immigration Act deprived wives of Commonwealth citizens settled in the UK by 1973 of the right to join spouses here and made them subject to the public funds test. Many Commonwealth men penalised by this change had worked for years in this country, but in an era of mass unemployment were unable to bring in family.

Conservatives put refusals 'beyond doubt'

Meanwhile an ongoing benefits curtailment strategy continued with regular initiatives to restrict access and occasional compensatory actions. In 1993 Urgent Case Payments – the basic safety net for many people from abroad – were restricted in scope. The government presented the change in inflammatory language, as ending 'an abuse' (Department of Social Security 1993). Their press release, *New Rules to Curb Abuse by People from Abroad,* quoted Social Security Minister Alistair Burt: 'We are determined to root out abuse of the welfare system and to put an urgent stop on this particular drain on the public purse'.

In fact, they removed a legal entitlement to temporary support for people in difficult circumstances, including people subject to the public funds requirement who were seeking to vary their leave. One such group was 'foreign spouses' who could previously claim urgent cases payments when applying for permanent leave at the end of the twelve-month probationary period. Women suffering domestic violence and relationship breakdown prior to 'regularising' their status, were left with no income to pay for places in refuges, causing extensive hardship. The Social Security Advisory Committee agreed not to comment formally on the regulation change or the hardships, in spite of its normal obligation. In a gross disregard of its obligations, it appears to have accepted the Government's view that the change reflected existing Home Office policy and that social security policy should be brought into line with this (Patterson 1993b: 16).

By 1993 too, a new question appeared on all income support claim forms, asking if people came to live in the United Kingdom under a sponsorship agreement. The incorrect impression was given that groups such as spouses would have no entitlement to benefits, even when given indefinite leave after a year. It was wrongly assumed that partners would have an ongoing duty to sponsor. In fact, only elderly dependants were sponsored with a specific 'undertaking' by families pledging ongoing support (Patterson 1993b: 17). Further changes in 1993 saw new law and guidance, stating that EC workseekers with 'no genuine chance of finding work' after six months on income support, may have to leave the UK, although there was no power to deport, and legal challenges were due. This guidance was later confirmed as unlawful in the House of Lords (*Remelien v. Secretary of State for Social Security and Another*, *Regina v. Same, Ex Parte Wolke*, *Times*, 1 December 1997).

The pattern of exclusionary policy-making contrasted with positive initiatives by the Benefits Agency (BA), which had been launched as a 'Next Steps' Agency in 1991, and had pursued objectives of the Citizen's Charter of 1992. It made efforts to act on national pledges on equal opportunities responsibilities, and to guarantee proper service for claimants whose first language was not English, and in 1993 launched guidance for staff, *Bridging the Language Barrier* (Patterson 1993a). These culture shifts led to improved local and national liaison, including regular national BA forums over future years, giving open settings to discuss and help shape BA 'operational matters', but not policy.

The new openness of the BA on equal opportunities and consultation in the early 1990s coincided with growing consumer assertiveness, strengthening rhetoric on inclusiveness under Prime Minister, John Major, and confidence in the opposition parties that electoral change was coming. Groups such as the Committee for Non Racist Benefits (1993) set out fresh charters advocating advances. A pattern continued though, of mitigating some of the harsher policies in practice, whilst incrementally more aggressive rhetoric, barely coded, and policy on social security was formulated by government.

The internal 'Lilley Reviews' of benefits were launched in 1993, leading to a series of cuts in benefits. Meanwhile, Home Office activities were influential with the Asylum and Immigration Appeals Act 1993 and a 'Scrutiny Review' of 'Inter-Agency Co-Operation on Illegal Immigration' announced later that year. In 1991, John Major had said, 'We must not be wide open to all-comers just because Rome, Paris and London are more attractive than Bombay or Algiers' (*Independent*, 29 June 1991).

The 1993 Act was pushed through with much talk of 'fraudulent' claimants and, amongst other changes, damaged the ability of minority ethnic families to maintain family links, by restricting the rights of visitors to the UK. The Home Secretary, Kenneth Clarke, gave cynical justifications in Parliament for a strict immigration control '. . . that our host population feels comfortable with', referring to potential 'terrible pressures . . . on our social services' if there was 'open entry' to people newly arrived (*Hansard*, 2 November 1992). An effect of the Act was to bring local authority housing staff more closely into the net of expected immigration interventions.

Announcing the scrutiny review, Home Secretary, Michael Howard said:

> . . . we should look afresh at ways in which Government as a whole – central and local – could co-operate more effectively to prevent abuse of the immigration laws and the drain on public funds which it often represents.
>
> (Home Office 1993)

Aims included improving efficiency and effectiveness of co-operation, extending guidance for staff and reviewing arrangements for exchanging information. The year 1994 saw early fruits of the scrutiny thinking, with special rules on 'persons from abroad' introduced into the Housing Benefit and Council Tax Benefit rules, forcing extensive local authority screening of claims.

One of the effects of the 1996 social security changes was to remove remaining entitlement to urgent case payments and housing benefit for appealing immigration decisions, or awaiting deportation or removal where the Secretary of State accepted it would be unsafe or unreasonable to take that action immediately (Child Poverty Action Group 1995). When announcing the cuts, the Government stated:

> Although there is no evidence that people are currently being paid benefit under these provisions, the Government intends to put beyond doubt its intention that those who have already received an immigration decision from the appropriate authorities should not be able to look to the benefits system for support during and after any appeal against that decision.
>
> (Department of Social Security 1995: 9)

Entitlement to disability benefits, child benefit and family credit was removed for all people with restricted immigration status in 1996, with these benefits added to the definition of public funds. Claiming public funds when disbarred was made a criminal offence. Temporary 'interim payments' were made harder to claim. New restrictions on sponsorship were implemented, with a single concession to take account of the death of some sponsors in the five-year period of non-entitlement, to make benefit payable. There were warnings of racist effects of the changes (Social Security Committee 1996: xii).

The benefit changes were presented as building on the 'Lilley Review' of benefits and the 'Scrutiny Review' by the Home Office, neither of which was public or published. From the scrutiny process, deep extensions of checks and ineligibility for several departments and agencies were announced (*Hansard*, 18 July 1995) and detailed guidance issued to local councils (Home Office 1996). In 1996 and 1997, the main restriction mechanisms from benefits were transferred wholesale into housing allocation and homelessness provisions. Whilst strongly opposing the changes, Shelter and the Commission for Racial Equality published guidelines for local authorities, urging the adoption of 'the least damaging practice in implementing these harsh pieces of legislation' (Shelter and Commission for Racial Equality 1997: 1). People left destitute because of immigration restrictions, or the habitual residence test (see below) were forced to survive by whatever means possible, through friends, charity or begging, whilst facing grave exploitation. Some found support from local authorities under the National Assistance Act 1948 or the Children Act 1989, but many local authorities placed obstacles in their path.

The 1996 changes marked the virtual death of the benefits safety net for people with restricted immigration status, save for those who retained transitional protection or support under limited reciprocal arrangements. Tiny numbers were also still entitled, in spite of the sponsorship rules, or briefly under disruption of funds from abroad. A further signal of the government's priorities in 1996 came with the abolition of its free social security helplines in minority ethnic languages, and the resources transferred over to new Fraud freelines, advertised nationally. The CRE concluded that a 'culture of suspicion' was the impact of internal immigration controls, rather than a culture of service. It found public officials and employers with dual, contradictory functions, staff unclear about their roles, delays, wrongful denials and unfair treatment (Commission for Racial Equality 1998), paralleling concerns of, for example, Amnesty International, who criticised the increased roles of low-ranking officials with no independent scrutiny (Cook 1998).

New Labour manoeuvres

The Labour Government abolished the disturbing 'Primary Purpose Rule' after taking office in 1997, but retained the 'probationary period' of one year before status could be changed and benefit entitlement claimed. It improved access with a 'concession' in 1999, allowing women leaving violent relationships, but without settled status, exceptional leave to remain on compassionate grounds. Award would lead to entitlements, but the level of proof of fear of violence was problematically high, and well above that required in other social provisions.

Proof required was 'an injunction, non-molestation or other protection order (other than an ex parte or interim order); or a relevant court conviction; and full details of a relevant police conviction' (*Hansard*, 16 June 1999).

New Labour's 1998 Green Paper reviewing social security, was silent on racial inequality and benefit barriers affecting minority ethnic communities. CNRB's submission of detailed evidence urging positive actions was ignored in the subsequent White Paper. Research concerns on racial inequality in benefits and the lack of ethnic monitoring, summarised by Law (1996: 51–80) and Craig (1999: 206–226), were also not addressed. One of the issues highlighted was the continuing injustice where women in polygamous marriages are denied widow's benefits (Committee for Non Racist Benefits 1998). Following a test case in 1997, Minister John Denham stated:

> The concept of marriage under British law is fundamentally monogamous. It would therefore be inappropriate to pay widow's benefit to widows, who, at the time of the death of their husbands, were in a polygamous marriage.
>
> (*Hansard*, 31 July 1997)

It is only with the Human Rights Act 1998, taking effect in 2000, that this issue is finally receiving serious scrutiny as a breach under the European Convention of Human Rights of the right to equal treatment in family life. This human rights focus allows belated recognition of minority ethnic communities with settled status, who should also benefit from government actions on child and pensioner poverty. For those subject to immigration control, challenges are likely to continue under the Human Rights Act for failure to make provision, and over adequacy of provision (Supperstone *et al.* 1999). The Race Relations (Amendment) Act 2000 brings new opportunities from April 2001, but affirms discrimination in immigration rules. Labour shortages led to first fledgling political endorsements of selective recruitment from abroad (*Guardian*, 12 September 2000), while from the European Commission there were moves to end the thirty-year rhetoric of 'zero immigration' (*Guardian*, 23 November 2000). However, the final nail in the coffin of UK social security for people with restricted status came with the abolition in benefit rules of the category of 'person from abroad' due to immigration status. It had been left as a lingering, void category, redundant in entitlements, its purpose served and overtaken by comprehensive disentitlement for those with restricted immigration status.

New presence and residence tests

Under the National Assistance Act 1948, simply being present in Britain was enough to qualify for benefit under the normal rules. Being present in Britain for a period is also now a condition of many non-contributory benefits. The DSS has long stated that a person must be lawfully as well as physically present, but the CPAG found no authority for this in a detailed summary of the law (Gurney 1993: 105). Case law on ordinary residence, another common condition, goes back at least to the 1920s and it is clear that immigration status does not determine this (Gurney 1993: 104). Social security commissioners read requirements of lawful presence and legal permission to work into the Social Security Act 1975 and regulations on 'availability for work', a condition that had been tied to immigration law in a Commissioner's Decision in 1957. On top of these disconcerting exclusions, two recent developments have resulted in further scrutiny and, indeed, attack on the protection of people arriving from abroad.

Presence and residence

The 1985 Green Paper *Reform of Social Security* included a plan for a new 'presence test' for Income Support, on the lines of the six or twelve months presence required for child benefit or mobility allowance. The *Daily Mail* had run a scare story 'Foreigners given free holidays' (21 August 1984), followed with 'Minister praises *Mail* for exposing the foreign scroungers – Holiday Racket stopped' (Child Poverty Action Group 1985: 12–13). EEC students were alleged to be 'seeking to leech on DHSS handouts', in a story which the CPAG proved to be inaccurate, with Government confirmation. Nevertheless, in justifying the proposed presence test, Social Security Minister, Tony Newton told the House of Commons Social Services Committee:

> . . . one of our anxieties in recent years has been the public anxiety that has been expressed on occasions – you will recall the controversy about students which has occurred once or twice – who are said to be able to get benefit which most people would not think reasonable that we should pay.

The proposed test contradicted EEC citizens' existing right to claim supplementary benefit – the precursor of income support (1988) and jobseekers' allowance (1996) – under normal rules and requirements for the first six months of their stay here. As such, the proposed test was likely to breach obligations under the Treaty of Rome. More extensively, the presence test 'would . . . have serious financial consequences for those immigrants from outside the Common Market . . . currently entitled to SB and [who] do not fall foul of the public funds test in the immigration rules' (Child Poverty Action Group 1985: 13). In the face of the Treaty of Rome breach and other opposition, the presence test was dropped in the 1986 White Paper.

Residence tests for non-contributory benefits were harmonised in 1992 at six months. Severe Disablement Allowance rules showed the greatest advance, down from a previous ten-year requirement. The rules still fell far short of the criticism of the CNRB, which called for abolition of the six-month rules in its 1993 charter, questioning for example, why child benefit should not be payable for any child newly living in the UK, or dependent on parents living here (Committee for Non Racist Benefits 1993).

Habitual residence

In August 1994 the 'Habitual Residence Test' was introduced for key means-tested benefits. The Government again justified the introduction of this test through an attack on 'Benefit Tourism' (European Union students coming to the UK for easy access to benefits) and through a brief, partly inaccurate, comparison with provision in other EU states (Social Security Advisory Committee 1994). The Social Security Advisory Committee advised not to implement the test, noting administrative difficulties and disproportionate effects on many minority ethnic communities. Echoing its criticisms of the previous extension of immigration restrictions to Housing Benefit, the committee noted that:

> . . . such a test has the potential to raise many . . . problems of discrimination . . . with the attendant risks of damaging community relations and deterring genuine claims from black and Asian British citizens.
>
> (Social Security Advisory Committee 1994: 11)

The opposition Labour Party opposed the test. The Government proceeded with it, with exemptions for refugees and EU workers. Moreover a lobby of Irish interests won a partial victory in that habitual residence in the 'Common Travel Area' of the UK and the Republic of Ireland, was introduced as a concession to pass the test. Intergovernmental concerns were crucial here, building on open access arrangements since the Ireland Act 1949. These political considerations led to a special accommodation on habitual residence which was not made available to members of other minority ethnic communities. Other discriminatory checks on Irish claimants in Britain, however, were set to continue (Patterson 1994).

The habitual residence test has had a disproportionate discriminatory effect on minority ethnic claimants. A NACAB report found that there was a strong correlation between those areas with large numbers of minority ethnic claimants and those with the largest numbers of people failing the test (NACAB 1996). Advice agencies in Birmingham and Yorkshire in 1997 reported that 90 per cent of their cases involving the test were minority ethnic claimants, whilst other agencies gave examples of unfairness, bias or overt racism in applying the test, in spite of national guidance urging fairness (Committee for Non Racist Benefits 1998). The test brought costly administration, gross inconsistency, lengthy advocacy and repeat applications. Its greatest effect has been to discourage applicants through refusals, discriminatory scrutiny and exclusion. With this organised hostility, many have not returned to challenge refusals, in spite of wrongful decisions or being likely to have entitlement soon, 'disappearing' from agencies, surviving harshly with unmet needs.

Local authorities administer the test for Housing Benefit claimants, and from 1996, for housing and homelessness applicants. One opportunity has been to influence them as independent decision-makers. For example, a Housing Benefit Office in a major city had refused over 100 claims, representing a quarter of all claims assessed under 'persons from abroad' rules, in the first ten months of applying the 1994 restrictions. As with most authorities, they had followed the harsh interpretation given in DSS national policy guidance to local authorities. Following representation by their welfare rights service, the council agreed to implement a more liberal interpretation, based on the Shah case and concerns on administrative burdens given by the government in their response to the SSAC. The refusals were reviewed and almost all who could be traced were reinstated on benefit. The *Shah* case (*R v. Barnet London Borough Council, Ex Parte Shah*, 1983) had defined 'ordinary residence' as being voluntarily in the UK for any settled purpose. This definition was eventually accepted, plus a requirement of 'an appreciable period of actual residence' (CIS 1067/95). The decision also confirmed that temporary absences would not breach previous habitual residence. However, some of the people hit hardest by the test were people long settled from the Indian subcontinent, who had returned from extended family visits in their country of origin.

The habitual residence test from 1994 had left a further anomaly in that EU migrant workers would satisfy the test, but British migrant workers returning from abroad were subject to the full test. A test case to the European Courts was finally resolved in 1999 in favour of a British national. The government used this occasion to end its two-year review of the test with a policy of deeming people returning to the UK after short or long periods of absence to be likely to pass the test. The new situation has eased the harshness of the test for people previously settled here, but maintained extensive refusals for new arrivals, including British nationals.

However the case law remains contradictory, with the *Swaddling* case in the European Court of Justice at odds with the *Nessa* decision in the House of Lords. One commissioner found on the earlier facts that 'such oddities are commonplace . . . [and] might indicate a need for amending legislation . . .' (CIS 3559/97). In 2001, benefit exclusion as a 'person from abroad' remains as a category due to failing the habitual residence test.

Treatment of asylum seekers

Treatment of asylum seekers has varied widely across countries, although since the mid 1980s a process of harmonisation has been developing at intergovernmental level in the EU. This process is characterised by convergence, restriction and secrecy (Joly *et al.* 1997: 22) and explored in depth elsewhere (Geddes 2000; Harvey 2000; Shah 2000). Governments have mattered, for example, the Conservatives refused to accept Chilean refugees in 1973, Labour organised admission from 1974, and the Conservatives ended the programme after their return to power in 1979.

Containment measures have been relentless. The UK introduced visa requirements for 85 countries by 1995, including all but two of the countries producing significant numbers of asylum applicants to the UK. Countries have included Sri Lanka in 1985, Sierra Leone in 1994 and Colombia in 1997. The Carriers Liability Act 1987 started a process of fines for travel companies bringing in undocumented passengers, and by 2000 P & O Stena was checking every lorry on entry (*Times*, 7 December 2000). Detention of asylum seekers has been higher in the UK than in any other European Union country. Family reunion rights have typically required four years' residence.

Settlement has lacked attempts at co-ordination until recently, but access to general benefits has allowed flexibility. However, Vietnamese refugees were dispersed in small groups in the UK under a programme in the early 1980s. Profiles have shown a pattern of difficult isolation, failing to take account of refugees' wishes to remain together as a community. Ten years later, the refugees had mostly regrouped in a few major cities.

Unequal social security

It is, however, the specific provision of social security for asylum seekers which I consider here. In the mid-1980s this consisted partly of Urgent Needs Allowances, paid for the first 14 days of claim with a 25 per cent reduction and no housing benefit, then rising to the standard supplementary benefit rate and housing benefit, but never including extra weekly payments for 'additional needs'. Alternatively, asylum seekers given temporary admission could claim ordinary supplementary benefit at the full rate. A British Refugee Council worker noted that:

> The DHSS rarely explain any of the . . . rules to the nonplussed refugees who may receive nothing or a totally inadequate amount to meet needs. There is no rational explanation for the fact that a newly arrived refugee who arrives in winter without any belongings, whose rent is £25 and who needs an overcoat and warm clothing receives either no payment at all while the matter is investigated, or a mere £22.50 for all his/her weekly expenses. But it's what the law says and the DHSS cannot pay for rent or clothes even if it wanted to.
> (Lane 1985: 12)

The 1988 benefit changes meant that most asylum seekers relied on the revised Urgent Cases Payments paid indefinitely at 90 per cent of the income support rate until their cases were resolved. With endless delays in making decisions on asylum, this often meant living below the poverty line for many years. The only 'premiums' payable were for pensioners. Minister Michael Portillo gave a wholly unsatisfactory justification of this policy:

> The reason for the abatement is that there would be no point in having rules which exclude people from benefit in certain situations if they could obtain full benefit by virtue of the urgent case rules.
> (*Hansard*, 20 July 1988)

There was partial respite in 1989 when other 'premiums' also became payable for people on urgent cases payments, following considerable campaigning. Political pressure mounted too for raising benefit to the full rate, but it was never developed.

In 1991 the Asylum Screening Unit was set up, amidst government and press talk of 'bogus refugees' and multiple claims for asylum, as the scene was prepared for a new Asylum Bill, and a General Election. Fraudulent benefit claims were exaggerated and remedies misdirected. Identity documents called 'Standard Acknowledgement Letters' (SAL) were introduced, but their issue was generally subject to delays of two to six months. Many BA offices adopted the attitude 'No SAL, no benefit', in spite of official policy to the contrary and alternative ways to confirm identity or status. Inaccurate guidance was issued to staff in 1992, and errors were reportedly made about decision-making authority, residence, time limits, previous documentation and form endorsements (Child Poverty Action Group 1992: 6). In 1993, the CPAG found that 'the difficulties and hurdles have since increased':

> It would appear that the Home Office are using their ability to delay the issuing of a SAL and the consequent delay in benefit payments in a punitive fashion . . . to penalise an asylum seeker for not entering the UK with a passport and visa documentation.
>
> (CPAG 1993: 7)

In 1986 there had been a vital recognition of the needs of asylum seekers, with new entitlement to 'single payments' – one-off grants – for clothing or furniture for asylum seekers and refuges. This successful arrangement was scrapped two years later with the introduction of the discretionary Social Fund. Resettlement for refugees was again undermined in 1992 when a court case on Social Fund grants found that a refugee could not be 're-establishing herself in the community' because she had lived all her life previously in Ethiopia (*R v. SFI, Ex Parte Amina Mohammed, Times*, 25 November 1992). This exclusion continued until 1998, when refugees who had received institutional care outside the UK could be considered for a discretionary grant. Families under exceptional pressures have also been able to apply for grants. However, the Social Fund has markedly failed to provide adequate help with clothing, or with essential furniture to allow refugees to set up home in the UK.

From disbelief to majority cuts

The early 1990s saw the further stepping up of a 'climate of disbelief' against asylum applications:

. . . the credibility and fairness of the Home Office's current determination policies and procedures is open to serious question. Along with other organisations working with refugees . . . the Refugee Council believes that 'a culture of disbelief' towards asylum seekers operates in the Asylum Division of the Home Office . . . many genuine applications are rejected and therefore the number of unfounded applications is exaggerated. . . . In the 18 months prior to the Act only 16% of applicants were refused either Refugee Status or Exceptional Leave to Remain. In the following two years some 80% of applications have been unsuccessful. This turnaround in the nature of decisions cannot be ascribed to any of the changes in the Act.

(Refugee Council 1995: 9–10)

The 1993 Act reduced the time allowed for appeals, reduced appeal rights for several groups, allowed fingerprinting and computer matching, and curtailed housing rights of asylum seekers, extending the scope of controls and discriminations to housing staff.

The withdrawal of all benefits in 1996 for the 70 per cent of asylum seekers who made their application 'in country' and for those pursuing appeals is well documented. It featured criticism by independent agencies, religious groups and the Social Security Advisory Committee (Social Security Committee 1996), widespread opposition and protests, desperate responses of local authorities and later narrow legal interpretations (Mynott 1999), a pliant media (Gabriel 1998), and extremely critical judicial interventions which gave brief respite (Justice *et al.* 1997). Expressing disbelief, the Court of Appeal found the policy of benefit withdrawal to be 'uncompromisingly draconian', 'inhumane', 'uncivilised' and illegal (*R v. SSHD, Ex Parte JCWI*, Court of Appeal judgment, 21 June 1996), but the cuts were quickly reintroduced through the Asylum and Immigration Act 1996.

Ministers had again talked of 'protecting the nation' and of 'people concocting stories about being political refugees'. Exploitation by organised groups was magnified and racialised to lend political cover to an unprecedented blanket response. In opposition, Shadow Home Secretary, Jack Straw pledged future withdrawal of these 'racialist laws' (*Guardian*, 27 November 1995), whilst in a ferocious assault, Shadow Social Security Spokesperson, Baroness Hollis said the Government was 'wilfully refusing to understand what it means to seek asylum and they are equally wilfully ignoring the advice of their own Social Security Committee' (*Guardian*, 5 February 1996)

Research reports soon found 'totally devastating effects of the benefit cuts' (Refugee Council 1996: 15), 'intense hardship', 'fraught . . . administrative problems' and a 'level of fear engendered' causing some people to avoid any contact with agencies altogether (Carter 1996: 1). The one conciliatory response by the government was to announce backdating of payments for people granted full refugee status, provided they claim within 28 days of the decision (Department of Social Security 1996). This 'concession', however, had minimal promotion by the authorities and low take-up. The standard letter from the Home Office on award of refugee status fails to mention the backdated entitlement. It also fails to advise unemployed refugees to claim Jobseekers' Allowance, resulting in loss of entitlement and erroneous overpayments. These errors, omissions and delays were repeatedly raised at the BA Refugee and Asylum Seekers Forum, with the Home Office relentlessly intransigent and the BA struggling to improve deficiencies.

Local authority interlude

The fall-back role for local authorities from 1996 followed early test cases and brought varied levels of responsiveness from Social Services Departments. It involved providing accommodation and meals for childless asylum seekers, or accommodation and cash support for families, but characterised by poor co-ordination and limited resources to develop services. Informal dispersal sought opportunistically to fill hard-to-let empty properties in the local authority and private sectors. Exploitative dispersal by southern authorities to private landlords in the north – unannounced and unprepared – sparked particular criticism (*Guardian*, 26 February 2000). Some local authorities brought a progressive desire for advocacy and improved standards. However, involvement was tempered by unwillingness to be given fundamental obligations under the emerging New Labour agenda, an issue discussed below.

Local authority staff responded positively to the task of dispersal arrangements for the Kosovar evacuees of 1999, and the wider climate was framed to encourage this. In Leeds, a wide partnership of social groups combined in giving a warm welcome and support (*Guardian*, 5 May 1999). A commentator on the Kosovo crisis, where human rights abuses and UK military involvement were highly visible, noted:

> Curiously, while the UK press has been generally unfavourable to asylum seekers and willing to run articles on 'bogus' asylum applicants, it has remained, in general, positive towards Kosovar asylum seekers.
>
> (Guild 2000: 83)

Involvement with other asylum seekers continued through a sub-sidised voluntary interim dispersal scheme of 1999. In the continuing pressurised role of dealing with everyday applicants there was some good practice, harnessing local good will. However, there was also much local opposition, often orchestrated by Press or politicians, and staff approaches and attitudes varied widely. When 58 Chinese people died tragically in a lorry, trying to enter the UK, a Social Services worker in a specialist reception team in a major receiving area was heard to say, 'That'll teach them a bloody lesson' (Interview with author, October 2000).

This 'worst case' example echoes the 1985 finding of DHSS staff, quoted above, and shows that enduring direct and institutional racism need continual challenge. The duties on services in local government gave fresh potential for more progressive attitudes, but the ad hoc, under-resourced responses failed to instil consistent, non-discriminatory treatment. The outcome was that local authorities took on secondary roles under the new arrangements from 2000, although still large providers of accommodation and active in local planning and advocacy.

Deterrence under New Labour

The brutality of the politics and arrangements inherited from the Conservatives gave Labour the chance to maintain the hostile language of 'deterrence', present themselves as 'sorting out the mess' and map an alternative path away from the straightforward, integrating measure of reinstating benefits. Moreover, by the international standards of recep-tion of asylum seekers, notably in poorer countries, provision of accommodation and assistance in kind was also possible, particularly for initial admissions (Justice *et al.* 1997). The 1998 White Paper, *Fairer, Faster, Firmer*, noted that

> . . . a significant number of EU countries provide accommodation and other support in kind. . . . At EU level, the Amsterdam Treaty provides for co-operation in the development of minimum stan-dards on the reception of asylum seekers.

The Government disingenuously argued the deterrent effect of in-kind support under the National Assistance Act (estimated at 15 per cent take-up) compared with benefits (estimated 85 per cent take-up). An assumption was that large numbers of asylum seekers would not take up in-kind support, relying on communities and families, preferably not arriving here at all. A no-choice national dispersal system was proposed, with in-kind provision, vouchers, and pocket money equivalent to 70 per cent of income support, plus heating and lighting. Major refugee organisations were contracted as referral points and a National Asylum Support Service (NASS) in the Home Office would co-ordinate contracts and decide on a test of destitution. The bias was to private accommodation providers and there were underdeveloped plans for regional multi-agency work. CNRB criticised the new isolated, seg-regated service with its likely insufficiencies and brutal consequences (*Independent*, 17 December 1998). The White Paper, however, also offered immediate respite for many thousands of people who had been waiting for years for an asylum decision, in a move to reduce the backlog.

The Immigration and Asylum Act 1999 is discussed elsewhere in this volume. The new system without benefits was implemented in 2000. The deterrent philosophy, poor planning and resourcing has meant that overcrowding, slum conditions, delays in vouchers, lack of local ser-vices, delays in local consortia and widespread racist attacks have been prevalent. For example, Hull became an early 'no referral' area in

> ... what appears to be a particularly hostile climate towards asylum seekers in the area. This follows a number of quite horrific inci-dents ranging from verbal and psychological harassment to extreme violence.
>
> (*Inter-Agency Partnership News*, September 2000: 3)

The Inter-Agency Partnership is the co-ordinating group of the vol-untary agencies implementing the 'One-Stop' offices and other aspects of the scheme. The 'One-Stop' staff have been positive and committed advocates for asylum seekers, but have strained under compromised pressures and conflicts of interest. Liverpool's 'One-Stop' office closed its doors to visitors in 2000, noting that:

> This system is not working. . . . Many do not receive travel vouch-ers enabling them to attend their all-important asylum interviews. . . . Many feel desperately unsafe or insecure in sub-standard accommodation. . . . NASS decision-making is unacceptably slow, and monitoring of local accommodation stan-dards has been poor. . . . The result is an unacceptably high level of racial harassment and attack . . . many victims may be afraid to go to the police. . . . NASS has not been able to meet their target of moving people within 7 days. Instead, move-on is taking 4–5 weeks . . . the numbers and pressure in our existing office

accommodation have become so great as to pose unacceptable health and safety risks to our clients and staff.

(*Refugee Action Chief Executive, Open Letter*, 31 October 2000)

In Nelson, Lancashire, Clearsprings, a private company reported as potentially making millions of pounds housing asylum seekers, was reported as using 'condemned slums' (*Observer*, 4 June 2000). A Manchester City Council report found 'evidence of terrible conditions, with some asylum seekers placed in boarded-up houses and others crammed several to a room' (*Manchester Metro News*, 22 September 2000). Glasgow City Council has signed a £100 million contract to take 2500 asylum seekers and dependants a year for five or six years. Other accommodation is also used. A local housing group has found extensive isolation and 'the fear of authority is such that many asylum seekers dare not complain about appalling living conditions for fear of deportation' (Qureshi 2001: 12).

The Disability Alliance claims that the government and NASS have failed to take the needs of disabled asylum seekers seriously (*Guardian*, 8 November 2000). With benefit entitlement removed in 1996, NASS from 2000 can meet exceptional needs, but could provide no single case of help given in the first six months (Refugee Council, correspondence with author, October 2000). After positive asylum decisions, access to benefit remains fraught with difficulties. New requirements for national insurance numbers have brought widespread delays, with temporary payments refused. Homelessness and destitution can follow from a positive decision on asylum, as well as from a negative one. Meanwhile, the Home Office's disastrous computer system was scrapped at a cost of £77 million (*Independent*, 15 February 2001). Widespread criticism has continued, for example, from the TUC, and with a national commission calling for cash support for asylum seekers at least at full income support level, free choice of available accommodation and an independent commission on all aspects of immigration, asylum and nationality (Commission on the Future of Multi-Ethnic Britain 2000). The UN has criticised the government's record on asylum and racial harassment, whilst welcoming its action plan on racially motivated crime (*Guardian*, 23 August 2000). Dispersal has failed to meet targets and a drift back to southern England is evident:

... the NASS-administered asylum support system as a whole is in crisis, and therefore in urgent need of reform . . . many of the problems now being encountered by both asylum applicants and

their advisers/representatives are precisely those that were widely –
and consistently – predicted by concerned organisations.

(NACAB 2000: 1)

The Minister ignored these pleas in noting that the system is 'in general,
working well' (Home Office 2000). A change in language from 'bogus' to
'abusive' asylum seekers has not removed the inherent provocation of its
presentation. A review of vouchers was due to report in 2001. There were
positive mentions of refugees' contributions and integration in construc-
tive, if lightweight, reports in 2000 (National Asylum Support Service
2000), whilst the European agenda considers standardising measures on
the treatment of applicants within the continuing negative framework
(Commission of the European Communities 2000). The elite nature of
policy-making in the EU has kept lobbying at that level specialised and
limited in effect (Geddes 2000). The UK government has led attempts to
dilute the Geneva Convention responsibilities on refugees (*Times*, 16
June 2000). The dominant agenda is of swift, cynical, perfunctory
refusals of asylum, with almost 40 per cent of decisions suddenly refused
in late 2000 on technical grounds of 'non-compliance' (*Guardian*, 26
January 2001). This means failing to meet a new rule of completing a
nineteen-page form in English inside ten days, noting too that dispersal
has seriously reduced access to legal advice (Amnesty International UK
2000: 50). Positive decisions on status in 2000 were down to 24 per cent,
with increased detention and accelerated funds aiming to quadruple
'removals' to 30 000 in 2001/2002. It is only the extreme rhetoric of the
Conservatives, pledging to lock up various categories of asylum seekers,
which gives the Government protection from wider condemnation.

Conclusion

In charting these chronologies of benefit disentitlements for people
coming to the UK from abroad, I have set out to show how policy has
been framed, challenged and implemented, and to explore effects on
claimants, communities and staff. The chronic detrimental effects of
benefit withdrawal for individuals and dependants with restricted immigration status cannot be over-stated. People left with nil income or
inadequate resources are intolerably poor, at extreme risk, denied basic
human rights. The fundamental principle of being able to survive safely
whilst, for example, appealing an immigration decision, has been ruthlessly discarded. The relentless negativity leads to people avoiding the
authorities, 'disappeared' from the system and left to survive in highly
exploitative settings.

Discrimination and hostility

The racially discriminatory treatment identified in the early 1980s has been bolstered by incremental benefit curtailments and the systematic extension of the immigration net into further social provisions. The immigration and identification checks have singled out minority ethnic communities for adverse treatment, errors and prejudice. The habitual residence test has added formal exclusions and increased racial disadvantage for people unaffected by immigration restrictions. It amounts to a new, disguised form of immigration control. The segregation of asylum seekers under a deterrence regime has been used cynically to inflame public hostility and has left many degraded. The security and rights of minority ethnic communities are thereby undermined (Faulks 2000: 143). A study of British citizenship found:

> The experience of minority ethnic groups is that they are on the one hand especially prone to exclusion through poverty, and on the other the basis of their social rights as citizens is suspect.
>
> (Dean and Melrose 1999: 147)

An effect of the successive changes has been increasingly to problematise minority ethnic groups within social provision, practice, the Press and public attitudes. The presentation of benefits and social policy has built on the rhetoric of immigration control, with sustained references to 'abuse', 'drain on the public purse', 'terrible pressures', 'public anxiety', 'bogus applicants', 'deterrence' and so on, pandering to perceived electoral attitudes of narrow sectoral groups. Immigration policy has overridden traditional welfare policy, with former entitlements presented as abuse and restrictive legislation trumpeted, even when negligible numbers are actually claiming:

> Although the press reports obsessively on those who are thought to be cheating the immigration authorities or the benefits agencies, there has been a striking dearth of information on the real situation of those legitimately seeking asylum and the subsequent outcome or on their mistreatment by officials in this country.
>
> (Alibhai-Brown 1999: 89)

It is unsurprising then, that recent opinion polls found greatly exaggerated perceptions of minority ethnic communities in Britain and falsely high assessments of asylum seekers' incomes (*Independent*, 23 October 2000). As a busy law centre has asked of a now-common local experience, 'How did *asylum seekers* become a term of abuse?' (South Manchester Law Centre 2000). Policy development has used extra structures within benefits, such as urgent case payments or special rules based on family membership, to legitimise reduced awards at below the poverty line. Justifications have been arbitrary or specific, on different occasions, but evidence of hardship and discrimination has been ruthlessly set aside. Informed debate is not sufficiently promoted, but as Spencer noted of local deprivation, 'government can act to stop immigrants and members of ethnic minorities being blamed' (Spencer 1994: 316). Indeed, there have been many positive actions by communities, advocates, staff and the wider public in support of asylum seekers and others from abroad, suggesting potential for much more humane policies.

Meanwhile Hansen's (2000) view of a liberal elite appears starkly at odds with the Conservatives' record, and over-generous to Labour's deterrence philosophy and closure of entitlements. As stopping trafficking and smuggling of refugees becomes a new endgame, the right of asylum in Europe is itself at risk (Morrison and Crosland 2000: 5). The 'firm but fair' rhetoric is used pervasively in social welfare provision, but the positive aspects remain limited, compromised or under-developed. This rhetoric has been further conflated in embracing the restrictive opportunities of the Europeanisation of immigration and asylum policy into so-called 'fairer, faster, firmer' futures.

Institutionalising exclusions

Successive staff groups and new organisational structures have been brought within the official net of immigration controls, adding scrutiny, errors and misconceptions to new refusals, relegating codes of non-discriminatory practice to a secondary role. Fresh energies have helped with advocacy, participation and commitment to welfare, but the wider framework is punitive, discriminatory and compromised. Services under severe pressure have delivered poorly. Legal challenges and opposition have had mitigating effects and added to the chorus of disapproval repeatedly shown in consultations on the restrictive developments in the UK. Advisers have used their experience and access to raise and profile concerns, whilst doggedly pursuing diminishing entitlements. The 'institutional spaces' notable in Geddes' (2000) approach have been widely pursued at a domestic level. However, protest has generally been channelled aside and refusals presented as fair. The slow turn to human rights arguments marks the likely way ahead. The fortress mentalities of politicians and policy-makers in the UK and the EU have succeeded for now in institutionalising exclusions from entitlements in the UK, racial discrimination and the 'culture of suspicion'. An emerging 'culture of expulsion' demands continual challenges for just provisions and human rights.

Acknowledgements

Thanks to Steve Cohen, Barbara Guest, Dean Herd, Jonathan Parr, and John Singh for comments. Thanks too to other correspondents. Responsibility for all views and details, however, is the author's alone.

References

Alibhai-Brown, Y. (1999) *True Colours: public attitudes to multiculturalism and the role of the government*, London: IPPR.

Amnesty International UK (2000) *UK Foreign and Asylum Policy: human rights audit*, London: Amnesty International.

Carter, M. (1996) *Poverty and Prejudice: a preliminary report on the withdrawal of benefit entitlement and the impact of the Asylum and Immigration Bill*, London: CRE and Refugee Council.

Castles, S. and Miller, M. J. (1998) *The Age of Migration: international population movements in the modern world*, 2nd edn, Basingstoke: Macmillan.

Chapletown CAB and Harehills and Chapeltown Law Centre (1983) *Immigrants and the Welfare State: a guide to your rights*, London: NACAB.

Child Poverty Action Group (1985) *Welfare Rights Bulletin 68*, London: CPAG.

—— (1986) *Welfare Rights Bulletin 73*, London: CPAG.

—— (1992) *Welfare Rights Bulletin 109*, London: CPAG.

—— (1993) *Welfare Rights Bulletin 114*, London: CPAG.

—— (1995) *Social Security (Persons from Abroad) Miscellaneous Amendment Regulations 1995, Submission to the Social Security Advisory Committee*, London: CPAG.

Commission for Racial Equality (1998) *A Culture of Suspicion, The Impact of Internal Immigration Controls*, London: CRE.

Commission of the European Communities (2000) *Proposal for Council Directive on Minimum Standards on Procedures in Member States for Granting and Withdrawing Refugee Status* 2000/0238 (CNS), Brussels: CEC.

Commission on the Future of Multi-Ethnic Britain (2000) *The Future of Multi-Ethnic Britain*, London: Profile Books.

Committee for Non Racist Benefits (1993) *Charter for Non-Racist Benefits*, London: CNRB.

—— (1998) *Time for Equality in Provision: a response to the government's green paper on welfare reform*, Manchester: CNRB.

Cook, D. (1998) 'Racism, immigration policy and welfare policing: the case of the Asylum and Immigration Act', in M. Lavalette, L. Penketh and C. Jones (eds) *Anti-Racism and Social Welfare*, Aldershot: Ashgate.

Craig, G. (1999) '"Race", social security and poverty', in J. Ditch, (ed.) *Introduction to Social Security: policies, benefits and poverty*, London: Routledge.

Dean, H. and Melrose, M. (1999) *Poverty, Riches and Social Citizenship*, London: Macmillan.

Department of Social Security (1993) *New Rules to Curb Abuse by People from Abroad*, Press Release 93/125, 13 July 1993, London: DSS.

——(1995) *Explanatory Memorandum to the Social Security Advisory Committee, Social Security (Persons from Abroad) Miscellaneous Amendment Regulations 1995*, London: DSS.

——(1996) *Peter Lilley Announces New Rule Bringing In Backdated Payments for Refugees*, Press Release 96/188, 24 September 1996, London: DSS.

Dummett, A. and Nichol, A. (1990) *Subjects, Citizens, Aliens and Others: nationality and immigration law*, London: Weidenfeld and Nicolson.

Faulks, K. (2000) *Citizenship*, London: Routledge.

Gabriel, J. (1998) *Whitewash, Racialised Politics and the Media*, London: Routledge.

Geddes, A. (2000) *Immigration and European integration: towards fortress Europe?*, Manchester: Manchester University Press.

Gordon, P. (1989) *Citizenship for Some? Race and government policy 1979–1989*, London: Runnymede Trust.

Gordon, P. and Newnham, A. (1985) *Passport to Benefits? Racism in social security*, London: CPAG and Runnymede Trust.

Guild, E. (2000) 'The United Kingdom: Kosovar Albanian refugees', in J. van Selm, (ed.) *Kosovo's Refugees in the European Union*, London: Pinter.

Gurney, J. (ed.) (1993) *Ethnic Minorities Benefits Handbook*, London: CPAG.

Hansen, R. (2000) *Citizenship and Immigration in Post-war Britain*, Oxford: Oxford University Press.

Harvey, C. (2000) *Seeking Asylum in the UK, Problems and Prospects*, London: Butterworths.

Home Office (1993) *Home Secretary announces study of inter-agency co-operation on illegal immigration*, Press Release 21/93, 13 October 1993.

——(1996) *Home Office Circular to Local Authorities in Great Britain: exchange of information with the Immigration and Nationality Directorate (IND) of the Home Office*, 24 October 1996.

——(2000) *Ministerial Statement*, STAT 028/2000, 22 September 2000.

Joly, D., Kelly, L. and Nettleton, C. (1997) *Refugees in Europe: the hostile new agenda*, London: Minority Rights International Group.

Justice, ILPA, ARC (1997) *Providing Protection: towards fair and effective asylum procedures*, London: Justice, ILPA, ARC.

Lane, D. (1985) *Refugees and SB*, in *Welfare Rights Bulletin* 68, London: CPAG.

Law, I. (1996) *Racism, Ethnicity and Social Policy*, London: Prentice Hall Harvester Wheatsheaf.

Layton-Henry, Z. (1992) *The Politics of Immigration*, Oxford: Blackwell.

Morrison, J. and Crosland, B. (2000) *The Trafficking and Smuggling of Refugees: the end game in European asylum policy?* UNHCR website.

Mynott, E. (1999) *Immigration, Asylum and the Provision of Services in Manchester: a preliminary report*, Manchester: Manchester Metropolitan University.

NACAB (1996) *Failing the Test*, London: NACAB.

—— (2000) *Support for Asylum Applicants, CAB Evidence*, London: NACAB.

National Asylum Support Service (2000) *Full and Equal Citizens: a strategy for the integration of refugees into the United Kingdom*, London: Home Office.

Patterson, T. (1993a) 'Time for equal access', in *Welfare Rights Bulletin* 114, London: CPAG.

—— (1993b) 'Racism and benefits', in *Advisor* 40, London: NACAB and Shelter.

—— (1994) *Claim in Vain? Social Security Benefits and the Irish in Britain*, Belfast: European Society for Irish Studies, Queens University.

Qureshi, R. (2001) 'Human Wrongs', *Roof*, 26(1), London: Shelter.

Refugee Council (1995) *The Social Security (Persons from Abroad) Miscellaneous Amendment Regulations 1995*, London: Refugee Council.

Shah, P. A. (2000) *Refugees, Race and the Legal Concept of Asylum in Britain*, London: Cavendish Publishing.

Shelter and Commission for Racial Equality (1997) *The Housing Act 1996 and the Asylum and Immigration Act 1996, Shelter and CRE Guidance on Eligible and Qualifying Persons*, London: Shelter and CRE.

Social Security Advisory Committee (1994) *The Income-related Benefits Schemes (Miscellaneous Amendments) (No. 3) Regulations 1994*, London: HMSO.

Social Security Committee (1996) *Benefits for Asylum Seekers*, HC81, London: HMSO.

South Manchester Law Centre (2000) *Defining our terms: how did 'asylum seeker' become a term of abuse?* Annual Report, Manchester: South Manchester Law Centre.

Spencer, I. (1997) *British Immigration Policy since 1939: the making of multi-racial Britain*, London: Routledge.

Spencer, S. (1994) 'The implications of immigration policy for race relations', in Spencer, S. *Strangers and Citizens: a positive approach to migrants and refugees*, London: IPPR/Rivers Oram Press.

Storey, H. (1986) 'United Kingdom immigration controls and the welfare state', in A. Dummett (1986) *Towards a Just Immigration Policy*, London: Cobden Trust.

Supperstone, M, Goudie, J. and Coppel, J. (1999) *Local Authorities and the Human Rights Act 1998*, London: Butterworths.

Titmuss, R. (1976) *Essays on 'The Welfare State'*, 3rd edn, London: George Allen & Unwin.

Part III
From theory to resistance

11 The 1999 Immigration and Asylum Act and how to challenge it

A legal view

Alison Harvey

Introduction

Sections 115–123 of the Immigration and Asylum Act 1999 (1999 Act) are grouped together within Part VI of that Act under a heading 'Exclusions'. They make provision for the systematic social exclusion of a free-standing category of 'persons under immigration control' as defined in Section 115(9) of that Act. Henceforth, those persons are excluded from the benefits system and from certain provisions of community care legislation that provide a safety net below that of benefits.

Support before the 1999 Act

Part VI of the 1999 Act is neither a new departure nor, necessarily, the culmination of the trend towards social exclusion. That immigration status should affect the support to which a person is entitled is nothing new. Some aspects of this are unsurprising: it has never been assumed that a holiday-maker could simply turn up at a benefits office and claim welfare benefits. The inclusion within the benefits system of those whose stay is of a longer duration, or of a different nature, has been gradually eroded. For leave to enter or remain to include a condition prohibiting any recourse to public funds has long been the rule rather than the exception. The Social Security Act 1986 made provision for 'persons from abroad' entitled to income support to receive 90 per cent of the applicable level of that benefit (the 'urgent cases' rate).

Since 1993, the pace of exclusion has increased. The Asylum and Immigration (Appeals) Act 1993 imposed a more restrictive definition of homelessness where asylum seekers were concerned. In 1996 a series of changes, culminating in the Asylum and Immigration Act 1996, excluded asylum seekers who did not claim asylum at the port of entry, but instead waited until they were inside the country to make a claim, from all entitlement to welfare benefits. The Housing Act 1996 further restricted the entitlements of people subject to immigration control under the homelessness legislation, and also prevented a local authority from giving a tenancy to these people. However, persons under immigration control were not excluded from community care legislation, as was established in a series of court decisions. Those who found themselves destitute as a result of the 1996 measures proved to be able to obtain support under the National Assistance Act 1948 and Children Act 1989.

The 1999 Act goes much further. However, as stated, it is not necessarily the culmination of the trend towards social exclusion. It does not tamper directly with the existing entitlements of persons under immigration control to health care, nor with that of their children to education and to the provisions of child protection legislation. Things could get much worse. Moreover there are more direct ways of effecting social exclusion. With the shortcomings and failures of the Part VI scheme becoming increasingly visible, the Conservative Party advocates a massive increase in the detention of asylum seekers. For those in detention, the issue of welfare support becomes a dead letter. Food, shelter, healthcare and education facilities are all provided (or not) through the mechanisms of the detention estate. Social exclusion is effected by barbed wire and the deprivation of liberty.

The debate in the UK to date has leapt straight from social exclusion to detention, but if human rights or financial considerations outlaw across-the-board detention there remains the possibility that 'reception centres', where powers to detain are not used, but where asylum seekers are forced to remain because they are denied food shelter, health care, education or anything else outside their walls, will become the focus of attention.

The 1999 Act

The 'Exclusions' provisions of Part VI come at the end of that Part of the 1999 Act, but logically they are where it begins. Those nine sections, shored up with a myriad range of statutory instruments covering such discrete issues as cold winter fuel payments, set about dismantling the rights of 'persons under immigration control', as defined therein, to benefits and to assistance under community care legislation.

The rest of Part VI is concerned with providing powers, not duties, to make alternative provision for some, although not all, of those excluded from mainstream provision. All duties to support a person 'subject to immigration control' are gone. Alternative provision is made for 'asylum seekers' as defined in Section 94, and for their dependants. Section 95 provides a power to support them. No alternative provision is made for others disentitled by the 'Exclusions' section. 'Asylum seekers' is a term of art within Part VI. It includes those who have made no claim for protection under the 1951 Convention relating to the Status of Refugees and its Optional Protocol of 1967. This is because it extends to those who have claimed the protection of the UK on the basis that their removal would breach Article 3 of the European Convention on Human Rights. This article states that 'No-one shall be subject to torture, inhuman or degrading treatment or punishment' and the jurisprudence of the European Court of Human Rights makes clear that this prohibits refoulement to a place where a person would face such treatment. The term 'asylum seekers' also includes those who have failed in their asylum claim, where they have children under 18, although in other contexts such people would no longer be considered asylum seekers.

More important are those excluded from the definition. An asylum applicant may be making a perfectly legitimate challenge, by way of judicial review, to the decision of the Immigration Appellate Authority to refuse to entertain his/her appeal against refusal of asylum. Such a person is not an 'asylum seeker' for the purposes of Part VI. Those whose asylum application has been refused, but who have outstanding representations before the Home Office asking them to reconsider, or to grant leave to enter or remain, are similarly not 'asylum seekers'. They are not entitled to support, however dilatory the Home Office may be in considering these representations. Support is also withdrawn from those whose claim fails, but who cannot be removed. Examples include situations where the Home Office is removing no-one to that country (e.g. in civil war situations where the airport is closed); where the individual cannot be documented for removal (certain governments, for example those of Algeria and China, have proved unco-operative in this respect); or simply where the Home Office has taken no steps to remove the person.

Quite aside from the definition, there are provisions for support to be terminated in certain circumstances, leaving the asylum seeker with no access to any support. As Earl Russell noted in the debates on the exclusion section in the House of Lords 'The Bill . . . clearly envisages that destitution may result and be unrelieved' (*Hansard*, House of Lords Report, 28 July 1999, col. 1576). One can see clear parallels with the government's proposals in the December 2000 Queen's Speech for legislation depriving those who have twice been convicted of benefits fraud to be denied any further access to benefits. Homelessness and starvation become new forms of punishment, meted out to those who are deemed to have transgressed the rules. Those who succeed in their claims are also at risk. Fourteen days after a positive decision, an asylum seeker loses entitlement to support, regardless of whether s/he has been able to access welfare benefits, or has even received the documentation from the Home Office enabling him/her to do this. This is most striking when a person without a dependent child under 18 has received news that his/her appeal against refusal of asylum has been allowed. It remains the responsibility of the Home Office to recognise that person as a refugee, and this can take months. Yet, 14 days after the decision on the appeal is received, support is terminated.

A separate system

Those who are to be supported receive this support under a wholly separate system. They do not fall under the Department of Social Security, or even local authorities (save under an interim scheme operating until Part VI is brought fully into force), but are instead the responsibility of a Home Office department, the National Asylum Support Service (NASS).

NASS determines whether or not the person is entitled to support, and what support should be provided. It contracts with others, including local authorities, private providers and certain voluntary agencies, to provide this support. The test of destitution used by NASS is a freestanding one. Similarly with the definition of what needs of the asylum seeker ('essential living needs') NASS is to meet, and with the definition of the standard of accommodation to be provided: the word 'adequate is used, rather than the term 'suitable', familiar from housing legislation.

The extent to which asylum seekers as defined are separated from mainstream welfare provision goes beyond even what is apparent on the face of the primary and secondary legislation. Welfare benefits provide a passport to various other kinds of support. In some cases, the NASS scheme effects similar passporting, but by no means in all. Thus for example, support from NASS does passport the supported person into free prescriptions, without the need to complete Form HC1, the form used for those on a low income, but not on benefits. However, it does not passport supported persons into receipt of free infant formula, or milk. Of course, the asylum seeker is excluded from the wide range of concessions available to those on income support, be it from educational establishments, rail or coach companies, or even recreational establishments, such as sports centres or theatres.

The government claims that children in NASS-supported families, while receiving accommodation and support for essential living needs from NASS, enjoy the full protection of the Children Acts in all other respects and the same rights as children as other children in the UK. However, this is far from straightforward. For example, NASS, in determining where the family is to live, will impact on the child's ability to access education. Similarly with other groups with special needs, NASS selects the accommodation. The location and standard of fixture and fittings in that accommodation, which may determine the supported person's safety, are determined by NASS.

Types of support

Part VI of the 1999 Act allows the government to control the form in which support is provided. Statutory instruments also make provision controlling the type of support. Further control is, of course, effected by NASS, a government department, having responsibility for the administration of the scheme. Part VI provided that support should not be wholly or mainly in cash. The Asylum Support Regulations 2000 make provision for each asylum seeker to receive £10 per week in cash, and prescribe the cash value of the total support each asylum seeker is to receive. The result is that asylum seekers receive the majority of their support in kind, or in vouchers, which can be spent at retail outfits that have entered into a contract with NASS. The means by which the support is to be delivered is regulated by NASS, by means of contractual arrangements with the direct providers.

A note on dispersal

Under the NASS scheme, it is intended that asylum seekers be dispersed away from London and the South-East, traditionally the areas where most of them have lived. London Boroughs and Kent had paid for asylum seekers out of their own pockets post-1996, when support was provided under the National Assistance Act and the Children Acts. Even when the government agreed to reimburse them for this, they still protested that they were taking the lion's share of the responsibility. They questioned the level at which they were reimbursed. They also noted that the reimbursement did not cover the hidden costs of health and education, nor, at the levels at which they were reimbursed, did it make it any easier for them to find low-cost accommodation for asylum seekers in the inflated rental markets of London and the South-East.

For these reasons, the NASS support scheme was to be a scheme of no-choice compulsory dispersal. NASS would dictate where in the country an asylum seeker was to live, with a statutory ban on taking into account the asylum seekers' preference. Normally, NASS would elect for areas outside London and the South-East. There is no doubt that this has further socially excluded asylum seekers. Many are sent to areas where no one speaks their language and from which their usual advocates, refugee community organisations, other refugee organisations, and asylum lawyers are absent. In many of these areas there is no history of work with asylum seekers and refugees, and thus the authorities in these areas have yet to embark, or are just starting to embark, on the steps that need to be taken to make services accessible to these groups.

The social exclusion of the destitute

Public pronouncements on the rationale for the separate system have varied over time. The government's White Paper 'Fairer Faster Firmer', and its 'Asylum Support: an information document' placed emphasis on the 'significant disincentive effect' NASS support was designed to have. It was separate, it was harsher, it would deter asylum seekers from coming here or, if they came, deter them from seeking state support. When the government found that this rationale was not proving as popular as it had been hoped, especially with its own back-benchers, who were concerned at the effect on children, it changed its tune. It argued that the scheme was one that would better suit persons under immigration control than a scheme predicated on social inclusion, because such people are different and have different needs. In the words of Lord Williams of Mostyn, 'our intention is to provide an intact scheme for those in that category [the category of "persons subject to immigration control"] in what I believe is a more responsive and sensitive way better suited to their needs' (*Hansard*, House of Lords Report, 28 July 1999, col. 1577).

The desire to deter asylum seekers from seeking state support sits ill with the rest of the scheme. Those who can support themselves or be supported by friends escape NASS. Those who can accommodate themselves can apply to NASS for support for essential living needs only. NASS will not go behind their statement of their accommodation provision, save insofar as is necessary to establish whether those who are accommodating them could also support them. It is not for NASS to consider whether the accommodation is overcrowded, or the children there are at risk. Such people escape dispersal, and of course, continue to use the health and education systems of London and the South-East.

Just how far at odds this is with the main scheme can be seen when one looks at work. If asylum seekers have no decision on their asylum application inside six months, they would normally be given permission to work, which is then withdrawn if they receive a negative decision on the asylum application. It is the government's aim that everyone should get a decision within six months – thus, that no one will work. The ban was similarly extended to volunteering. Later, when the ban on volunteering was removed, nonetheless the conditions imposed on volunteering were by any standards extraordinary. Letters sent out by Rachel Reynolds of NASS in early 2000 made reference to NASS guidance that stated, inter alia:

> Unless unavoidable for cultural or religious reasons, meals should not be provided by voluntary organisations as they might be construed as a wage in kind. . . . Potentially ambiguous situations in which a volunteer was reimbursed for travel which he/she would have undertaken anyway (e.g. reimbursement for travelling to a volunteering venue once a week on the volunteer's normal shopping route) should be avoided.

Enforcing social exclusion

Support 'available or reasonably expected to be available' to an asylum seeker, including from voluntary bodies, can be taken into account in assessing what level of support should be provided to a person. Thus a charity, or indeed an individual, is forced to accept the government's definition of what is essential to the asylum seeker. If they seek to top this up NASS can reduce the asylum seeker's support accordingly. Given that travel, toys and recreational activities are all excluded from the definition of essential living needs (see Reg. 9(4) of the Asylum Support Regulations 2000, SI 200/704), it is clear that this definition is very unlikely to be shared by the asylum seekers, charities, and charitable individuals on whom it is imposed. The government itself struggles with how far it will press the definition of essential living needs. Faced with an outcry on the exclusion of toys, it agreed that a child could be given a toy without support being reduced. However, it has failed to give any coherent explanation of how this fits with the rationale for the scheme, or what the implications might be for other types of support – household goods or money – that charities might wish to provide.

The scheme in practice

The creation of a Home Office department that would fulfil many of the functions of the welfare state, and towards a diverse and very vulnerable group of recipients, is to say the least an ambitious exercise. The social engineering involved in dispersal is also ambitious. To these must be added the experiment of providing support in kind or in vouchers.

One stated government aim was that the scheme should be protected from legal challenge. The government representative in the Special Standing Committee which examined the Bill in the House of Commons, Mike O'Brien, Under-Secretary of State in the Home Department, made this explicit. This is demonstrated by his statements on particular clauses:

> If we allow things to remain the way they are, all sorts of legal challenges may be mounted under the Children Act . . . to undermine the way in which the Asylum Support Directorate provides accommodation in particular areas, offers financial support and operates the dispersal policy.
>
> (Debate on then clause 99, *Hansard*,
> House of Commons Report, Official Report of the Special
> Standing Committee, Asylum and Immigration Bill,
> Twentieth Sitting, 11 May 1999 (Part II), col. 1465).

> Everything would be subject to judicial review. The state would have to be far more careful about decisions to offer accommodation and take much greater care in its analysis of circumstances.
>
> (Debate on then clause 74, *Hansard*, House of
> Commons Report, Official Report of the Special
> Standing Committee, Asylum and Immigration Bill,
> Nineteenth Sitting, 4 May 1999 (Part I), col. 1299)

There was little or no focus on the world outside the courtroom. There was little or no focus on the asylum seeker caught up in the scheme; the attention was on those who would be deterred from coming to the UK because of it. That an asylum seeker faced with no-choice dispersal might prefer support in kind to a London address that was little more than a *poste restante*, was not considered. That asylum seekers would not be able to live if the definition of essential living needs did not correspond to those needs they had, was also not a consideration. That persons would remain in need of food and shelter despite no longer being entitled to support, was not taken into consideration. In short, reality was firmly excluded.

From the point of view of the human misery created by the scheme, and the wider social problems entailed by the efforts of asylum seekers to find other ways to survive, these issues are central. From the point of view of the administrative efficiency of NASS, their importance is more difficult to determine. The asylum seekers' inability to eat properly or to live in safe accommodation will in many cases never be visible to the NASS bureaucracy. Little attention has been given to the wider effects of the scheme. Among the questions that remain to be answered is whether more asylum seekers are working without permission, in order to meet their true 'essential living needs'. If so, are they exploited by unscrupulous employers? Are they exploited for prostitution? Is working without permission lining the pockets of those who exploit immigrants, and thus fuelling the very trafficking of persons to engage in illegal employment that the government wishes to stop? Are asylum seekers staying outside the scheme by living in overcrowded accommodation that breaches health and safety legislation and puts children and others at risk?

Surprisingly, equally little attention has been given by government to the effects of the scheme on their own ability to determine the asylum application. As the Bill that became the 1999 Act progressed through parliament some consensus emerged that faster decision making lay at the heart of reform of the asylum system. A short turnaround time for applications gave the would-be economic migrant and any traffickers profiting from his/her presence little opportunity to earn money in the UK, and, coupled with prompt removal of those whose claims did not succeed, could reasonably be expected to make the country a less attractive destination to those not in need of protection from persecution. Yet at many levels the NASS scheme appears to militate against the 'faster' system desired by government. Enormous administrative difficulties have arisen in attempting to relay dispersed asylum seekers to London for interviews and appeals. They are far from lawyers who could assist them in presenting their claims, and may be far from anyone who can even translate the letters explaining what is expected of them. Cases drag on because during the period when an initial statement of the application was desired, the asylum seeker was grappling with applications for support and dispersal and had no access to any means of presenting a coherent application. The lack of any support at the end of the process does not merely leave the failed asylum seeker with little or no incentive to remain in contact with the authorities and thus to be available for removal; by depriving the asylum seeker of an address or any support whatsoever it can make continued contact quite impossible.

Even without any exploration of these wider issues, it is manifestly clear that the scheme in practice is not functioning as it was intended to do. Many more applications for support only than for support and accommodation have been received, thus dispersal is not working. During the passage of the Bill, officials spoke of an intention that NASS should determine applications for support within hours. Dispersal was to follow swiftly. By the time the Asylum Support Regulations 2000 were promulgated, NASS was intending to make the majority of decisions within two days, to a maximum of one week, and then to disperse swiftly. Instead, it is taking months to determine an application. Asylum seekers awaiting a decision on their application or a dispersal address are accommodated by certain voluntary organisations which have contracted with NASS. The asylum seeker receives support in kind only, no cash or vouchers. S/he cannot travel at all and is left virtually helpless. The log-jam in the emergency accommodation has overwhelmed the voluntary organisations involved.

As to dispersal, the theory was that asylum seekers would be dispersed in mutually supportive clusters of sizeable groups of individuals speaking the same language or from the same countries, and placed in areas where services were available or would quickly become available to them. This has not happened. Dispersal was also predicated on a model of supported housing, whereby the housing provider would be responsible for putting those housed in touch with GPs, lawyers and other services. But the terms of the contract impose only a limited responsibility, and the majority of the housing providers have no experience of supported housing, nor any particular interest in it.

Most striking as the scheme has progressed is its relationship with the welfare state. Not with the benefits system, as there asylum seekers are excluded, but with local authorities. One of the initial aims of the support scheme was to relieve local authorities of their responsibilities towards asylum seekers. As the design of the scheme progressed it became increasingly clear to NASS that it would be unable to function without the support of local authorities. It conceived a desire to contract as much accommodation as possible from local authorities, and to look to them for other services. The Local Government Association, no doubt convinced that any problems with the scheme would come home to local authorities to roost, and lobbied by authorities in London and Kent, were initially co-operative. However, as authorities throughout the country entered into detailed negotiations with NASS, it became increasingly clear to them that they would receive little in exchange for their co-operation. The result was that NASS has ended up contracting with private providers for the majority of the accommodation it needed, while increasingly turning to local authorities to provide services it is unable or unwilling to deliver. Thus, for example, it has looked to loopholes in the legislation to ensure that local authorities assess those with a disability and provide the services and support that these people need. One of the hardest fought provisions of the 'Exclusions' section was that of exclusion from the provisions of the Children Act 1989 and equivalent provisions for Scotland and Northern Ireland. Early drafts of what is now Section 122 excluded children in asylum-seeking families from the provisions of the Children Acts. This proved unpopular. The compromise finally reached reflects the ambiguous relationship between NASS and local authorities. Where an asylum-seeking family is entitled to NASS support, the Secretary of State must provide it. In these circumstances, a local authority may not provide assistance under the Children Acts, with assistance narrowly defined as the provision of accommodation or support for essential living needs. Local authorities can thus be required to top up NASS support, for example by providing school uniforms or covering the cost of travel to school. However, if the family loses its entitlement to NASS support, for example because it breaks the conditions on which support is provided, then responsibility for supporting the family falls to the local authority within whose area the family is living, the latter condition inserted to preserve the dispersal arrangements. Thus, far from being relieved of the responsibility for the support of asylum seekers, local authorities are made responsible for those who have proved to be NASS's most difficult clients. In practice, the notion of a separate system has been considerably eroded.

Challenging the scheme

There is every sign that the NASS scheme is perfectly capable of self-destructing, and that only the efforts of local authorities and certain voluntary organisations who entered into contractual relationships with NASS to deliver some of its services, are holding it together. If they pulled out, there is doubt that the scheme could survive. But, as is common when the choice is between revolution and reform, the effects of a sudden collapse of the system on those whom NASS is now supporting, together with the many facets of the contracts between NASS and the voluntary organisations, have deterred them from seeking to deal it a deathblow.

There are, broadly speaking, three ways of challenging Part VI before the law. First and most satisfactory, are challenges that limit the scope of the exclusions from welfare support. Second are those challenges that attempt to reduce the class of those with no entitlements whatsoever to support, by bringing them within the scope of the alternative, NASS, support scheme. Third, there are ways of challenging the operation of either the exclusions or the NASS scheme. All these challenges may have the character of reforms, mitigating the worst effects of the social exclusion, but contain within them the potential to strike at the heart of the project of social exclusion, by taking people outside the NASS scheme and into mainstream support, by overburdening NASS, by overburdening others so that support for NASS is undermined, and generally making the scheme unworkable.

Challenging exclusion from the welfare state

Provisions of European legislation provide one challenge. Nationals of states which have ratified the European Social Charter, or of states which have entered into association agreements or other reciprocal agreements with states of the European Economic Area, are entitled to certain welfare benefits in certain circumstances. While domestic provisions offered more favourable support for the majority of those whose states had ratified, these provisions were little used, but with NASS support as the alternative, it has become worthwhile to explore how far they can be used.

The 'Exclusions' section of Part VI was modified, due to pressure during the passage of the Bill, so that exclusions from community care legislation were limited in scope. Only when the needs of the person under immigration control arise solely from destitution or the physical effects of destitution, is the asylum seeker excluded from the provisions of the National Assistance Act 1948, the Health Services and Public Health Act 1968, the National Health Service Act 1977, and equivalent provisions for Scotland and Northern Ireland, and other similar legislation. In the case of *R v. Wandsworth Borough Council, Ex Parte O and R v. Leicester City Council, Ex Parte Bhikha* [2000] 4 All ER 590 (CA), [2000] 1 WLR 2539, the government, intervening, sought to argue that the needs of a person for food and shelter arose from destitution, albeit that the person was suffering from an illness, or had a disability or disorder. The Court of Appeal preferred the appellants' construction of the legislation: 'if an applicant's need for care and attention is to any material extent made more acute by some circumstance other than mere lack of accommodation and funds, then, despite being subject to immigration control, he qualifies for assistance. Other relevant circumstances include, of course, age, illness and disability'. Lord Justice Simon Brown observed, 'if there are to be immigrant beggars on our streets, then let them at least not be ill, old or disabled'. This opens the door to bringing a wide range of people within community care support. The case of 'O' concerned persons under immigration control who were not asylum seekers and thus never had any right to alternative provision. Another group likely to benefit from the effects of the legislation are failed asylum seekers, whose entitlement to alternative provision has ceased. The provisions also provide a route by which groups with special needs can be supported. Following the judgement of the Court of Appeal in Westminster City Council v NASS (2001) EWCA CIV 512, C/2001/0596, such persons can be supported entirely under the provisions of community care legislation, and not by NASS at all. It might be expected that representatives of such asylum seekers would be those arguing for such an interpretation. However, overwhelmed and under-resourced, and facing severe criticism for its treatment of these groups, NASS itself found off-loading this group onto social services more attractive than maintaining its programme of a separate system of support.

It seems unlikely that a lawyer is going to find any single provision of any act to drive a coach and horses through the 1999 Act in the way that the National Assistance Act 1948 drove a coach and horses through the 1996 legislation. However, there remains the potential to identify existing legislation, from which certain groups of asylum seekers have not been excluded by the exclusions provisions of Part VI, that will benefit members of those groups. For example, Section 24 of the Children Act 1989 is untouched by the exclusions provisions. This section allows a local authority to accommodate and provide cash to a person turning eighteen who was in a UK children's home or looked after by any local authority when aged sixteen or seventeen. Such support can be provided until the young person is twenty-one. The 'Exclusions' section of Part VI is no way affects this entitlement, and a young person so supported would never come into contact with the NASS scheme, because s/he would not be destitute. The barriers to the use of this section to support asylum seekers are not legal ones, but practical and financial ones. A local authority will not be reimbursed by the government for expenditure under Section 24, which provides a huge disincentive to its using its powers in this way.

There will be cases in which the very harshness of the support arrangements (or lack of same) attached to a particular immigration status may provide an argument for seeking to get that status changed. As described above, a person whose asylum claim has failed, but who cannot be removed, is not entitled to any NASS support whatsoever. Where for example, the person is not being removed because a civil war has meant that the Home Office are not removing anyone to that country, then the destitution the client faces strengthens the argument that the Home Office should grant the person Exceptional Leave to Remain for a limited period.

Similarly, the harshness of the support system may strengthen the hand of those attempting to challenge the Home Office where it is being dilatory. Where for example, an asylum application has failed, but there are representations outstanding before the Home Office that the asylum seeker should be granted leave to remain on some other basis, it may be possible to force the Home Office to speed up consideration of those representations.

Extending the ambit of the NASS scheme

As noted above, the support scheme appears to have been conceived with little regard for the determination of the claim for asylum. The problems may go further, in that they may ultimately affect the way in which a claim is presented. If a person alleges that removal will breach Article 3 of the European Convention on Human Rights, s/he is an asylum seeker within the definition of the NASS scheme. There is thus every incentive to make such a claim. Nor will it necessarily be difficult to phrase a wide range of arguments that a person cannot be returned in terms of Article 3. Article 3 prohibits torture, but also inhuman or degrading treatment or punishment. The person with AIDS, who argues that there is no treatment available in the country to which return is proposed, can argue that return in such circumstances would constitute inhuman or degrading treatment. The person in whose country a civil war rages, can frame a similar argument. The person who fears violence, but for private reasons, not the reasons of race, religion, nationality, political opinion or membership of a social group, may also look to Article 3. It is also likely that claims will be made under this article where removal would separate a person from family members. Such claims would more naturally be brought under Article 8 ECHR (right to private and family life) and would undoubtedly have more chance of success under that article. But what matters for the purposes of Part VI support is not whether the Article 3 claim is ultimately successful, or indeed well-founded, but whether it has been made at all. Similarly with making a fresh claim for asylum, or with making a claim at all. Part VI provides a new incentive for doing so.

Where legal challenges to a NASS decision are brought, it may be possible to seek interlocutory relief that will oblige NASS to continue to support the asylum seeker. Similarly, where legal challenges to the decision on the asylum claim are brought, it may be possible to seek interlocutory orders which would then have the effect of ensuring that the appellant remained an asylum seeker for the purposes of the definitions used in Part VI. Representatives will argue that the judges of the High Court must either expedite the case before them, or else grant interlocutory relief. It seems unlikely that the High Court would be in a position to expedite all of the claims relating both to asylum applications and to asylum support that are brought before it.

Other ways of ensuring inclusion in the NASS scheme fall clearly outside the scope of 'legal challenges', albeit that they are perfectly legal. Given that those with dependent children under eighteen are entitled to support until removal, an asylum seeker who has a child or undertakes parental responsibility for a child, thereby alters his/her entitlement to support.

Challenges to the operation of the NASS scheme

As described above, the government sought to protect the Part VI support scheme from legal challenges. The choice to provide powers rather than duties to support asylum seekers, statutory prohibitions on taking into account the preferences of an asylum seeker as to accommodation, statutory definitions of what makes accommodation adequate, were all designed to achieve this. In short, all was done to seek to protect the system from judicial review, save that which would have made a difference: the provision of sufficient support so that the asylum seeker had no legitimate cause for complaint. In these circumstances and given the severity of the provisions of Part VI, the scope for judicial review remains enormous.

A powerful tool for use against Part VI is undoubtedly the Human Rights Act. Whether or not withdrawal of all entitlements to food and shelter will be found to breach Articles 2 and 3 of the European Convention on Human Rights, when coupled with the prohibition on discrimination in respect of the rights protected, it becomes difficult to square Part VI with obligations under the Human Rights Act. Dispersal far from family members or from support networks also has implications for rights under Article 8 of the European Convention on Human Rights, which protects rights to private and family life.

However, the Human Rights Act is not the sole tool available to lawyers. The challenge to the legal profession is to exploit all the legislation designed to promote social inclusion to fight the social exclusion set in train by Part VI. Issues of environmental health, of the rights of the disabled, of obligations towards children, including providing them with an education, can all be used to found legal challenges. Will the accommodation provided by NASS satisfy the full rigours of child protection legislation, or the requirements of legislation designed to protect the disabled and their rights? Vouchers are issued to the head of the family, normally a man. Is this acceptable under sex discrimination legislation? Vouchers are issued solely to asylum seekers or their dependants, and bear their names. They pass from the asylum seeker to the retailer accepting them. Does this breach the Home Office undertakings of confidentiality towards asylum seekers?

Challenges to the support system provide a test of our commitment to the Human Rights Act 1998 and of the strength and scope of our social welfare legislation and the extent to which it protects vulnerable groups from mistreatment or exploitation, public health, and the rights of individuals and minorities. Is it so very easy to circumvent or can its ability to tackle the NASS system reveal it to have powers to protect all within the territory, powers which can then be used for the benefit of all within the territory, not only persons under immigration control?

12 Fair immigration controls – or none at all?

Beth Humphries

Introduction

It is a commonsense notion that we must have immigration controls of some sort, since Britain is a small and overcrowded island. Controls must be fair, it is argued, and should treat all people equally. Many who oppose this position and advocate no immigration controls, take apparently rational positions to refute the arguments (Britain is not overcrowded; there are more people leaving than arriving annually; immigrants have enhanced the British economy and culture, and so on). In this chapter, I examine both the case for 'fair' immigration control and the arguments entailed in anti-immigration control positions. I argue that it is not possible to make an unfair system fair, but that many of the contrary arguments do not enhance the case against immigration controls. Indeed they make unintended concessions to those who advocate controls.

Making an unfair system 'fair'

Writers such as Carens (1987), Dummett and Nicol (1990) and Spencer (1994a, b), and organisations such as the Stonewall Immigration Group (2000), illustrate the arguments offered for a 'fair' system of immigration controls. Carens argues that borders should generally be open, with people normally free to leave their country of origin and settle in another, subject only to the constraints that bind current citizens in their new country. However, if migrants came in very large numbers, according to Carens, restrictions on entry would be justified to preserve public order.

Dummett and Nichol agree with Carens's position on freedom of movement explicitly, and implicitly in their reference to the potential problem of 'massive' immigration where the resident population's culture could not be maintained, or where the immigrants, though few in number, 'actively destroy it' (Dummett and Nichol 1990: 276). But who is to be the arbiter of 'massive' immigration, or of whether a 'culture' is being 'destroyed'? Such language has not been employed in the case of the principle of freedom of movement within the European Community. This freedom includes not only movement of labour, but also a worker's spouse, children, dependent parents or grandparents, regardless of their nationality. The British experience suggests that 'massive' and 'hoards' and 'destruction of the culture' enter immigration discourse very readily when those seeking entry are constructed as undesirable, which has focused on different groups at different historical moments, and currently targets those who are black and poor or Muslim, or Roma (Hayter 2000). The construction is not applied in the case of white people from rich countries. And 'culture' implies a homogeneous mono-cultural society that one would be hard-pressed to find anywhere in the world. This 'imagined community' is brought into play to reinforce the idea of the threat that foreigners and aliens bring to the stable and established society. It is of interest that the target of these policies is 'aliens', since Community law imposes a duty on member states to admit their own nationals, even if they are criminal, poor, diseased or engaged in international terrorism. Those who argue for 'fair' immigration controls tacitly reinforce this nationalist and racist stance, even when their motives are liberal.

With regard to the general principle, Dummett and Nicol say that an individual may have an acknowledged personal right of some kind, but the way the person uses that right is subject to moral limits, and may be limited by law. They argue that

> . . . one may assess the way a state uses its acknowledged discretion on the admission of aliens as 'just' or 'unjust' according to the general principles of law and the standards set by international agreements.
>
> (Dummett and Nichol 1990: 263)

Spencer (1994a) supports this position, and her edited publication *Strangers and Citizens* is possibly the most important recent UK publication advocating 'fair' immigration controls. It is published jointly by Rivers Oram Press and IPPR (Institute for Public Policy Research), an organisation closely associated with the Labour Party and with trade union research and policy. It was established in 1988 'to provide an alternative to the free market think tanks' (Spencer 1994b: xiii). Sarah Spencer is a research fellow at IPPR. The book is the result of a series of seminars hosted by IPPR, and represents the organisation's recommendations to the British Government, for an approach to fair immigration and refugee policy. An examination of it reveals the contradictions that arise as a result of efforts to describe this fair policy. It takes the position that purely humanitarian grounds cannot alone form the basis of a sound immigration policy, and the overall argument is towards economic factors as the main criteria informing policy. Although it calls for 'objective research' about the skills and occupational groups required, it also acknowledges that 'the social context is critical to whether immigration is perceived to be of economic benefit' (Spencer 1994a: 11). This is a reference to stereotypes of immigrants as 'scroungers' of one sort or another, but the sentence also implies that the ways economic needs are *defined*, results in the exclusion of people with particular skills. A flaw of *Strangers and Citizens* is that, in spite of this admission, it then pursues the economic argument as though a country's economic needs are always obvious, uncontested and uninfluenced by 'the cultural context'.

Findlay, one of the contributors, compares North America with western Europe, arguing that the USA and Canada are more welcoming of immigrants because of a positive multi-cultural vision, while in western Europe resistance to multi-culturalism is strong. He makes the point that 'cultural factors produce different interpretations of what is meant by the economic costs and benefits of migration' (Spencer 1994a: 166), yet neither he nor any of the other contributors, follows through the conclusions of this. When Spencer calls for 'research' (Spencer 1994a: 312, 320, 329, 330, 343), and 'factual evidence' (Spencer 1994a: 345), she also needs to acknowledge that research does not take place in a vacuum – the 'view from nowhere' – but is located in the interests, ideologies and motives of dominant groups. The kinds of answer that research produces, depend on the kinds of question it asks. Both Zimmerman's (1994) statistical analysis, and the volume brought together by Harnisch *et al.* (1998), confirm that the demand for unskilled and low-paid jobs is usually defined in terms of immigrant labour, and that immigrants tend to be 'substitutes for low-qualified natives' (Zimmerman 1994: 54). Indeed, when European home affairs ministers discussed the issue of 'replacement migration' Summer 2000, the French interior minister questioned the basis of the figures presented and denounced proposals to accelerate immigration as an employers' tool to try to depress wages (*Guardian*, 30 October 2000: 17).

The attempt to define 'fair' immigration controls leads to other muddled arguments. Spencer's book considers the labour market impact of immigrants, implications for housing, and the balance between taxes and costs they incur in education, welfare and health services, and says that research in other countries does not support the belief that immigrants are a drain on public resources. Yet the apparently supportive argument that it is in the country's interest to assist newcomers in English language skills and employment training (Spencer 1994a: 331), suggests that an investment of public resources _is_ needed. Similarly, it is argued, 'common sense would suggest that two parent families are more likely to earn enough to be self-supporting than single parent families where one spouse is excluded from the UK' (Spencer 1994a: 331). Although presumably the intention here is to make a case to allow both parents entry to the UK, it may also be used to exclude the entire family. The point being made here is that the linguistic contortions necessary to support 'fair' controls can lead to outcomes unintended by the authors.

The recommendations of _Strangers and Citizens_ are prefaced by the injunction that controls should be non-discriminatory, fair and clear. The book deplores the notion that it is possible to identify safe countries from which no application for asylum could be legitimate, arguing that this breaches the principle of self-determination of each case and ignores the reality that there may always be exceptional circumstances (Spencer 1994a: 334). At the same time, there is approval of the view that those conducting interviews should be well informed about the applicants' country of origin, 'and thus in a position to assess the veracity of their persecution claim' (Spencer 1994a: 333). This is seen to improve both fairness and efficiency of the asylum procedure. This contradiction demonstrates the impossibility of replacing the discretion, and therefore the prejudices of immigration officers, with 'factual evidence' as argued by Spencer elsewhere.

Although _Strangers and Citizens_ deplores racism and discrimination against both minority ethnic residents and would-be immigrants, in a number of ways it reinforces discriminatory practices. For example, on very uncertain evidence, it predicts 'mass migration on an unprecedented scale' (Spencer 1994a: 322), thus justifying its argument for the necessity of border controls (and incidentally using highly charged language which can be and has been, used against minority ethnic residents). Spencer's view that 'government has the right to put the interests of its existing residents, including members of ethnic minorities, before those of individuals who want to settle here' (Spencer 1994a: 319), is naïve, given the evidence of the impact of internal controls on black communities (Hayes 2000 and this volume). Her faith in race relations legislation (Spencer 1994a: 319) as an effective means to counter racism is also misplaced. This tendency to pander to discriminatory beliefs is reinforced by the opinion that the UK is unlikely, 'even in the longer term', to need substantial numbers of migrants to fill labour shortages (Spencer 1994a: 330). There is also approval of the practice of investigating marriages to ensure they are genuine, and of DNA testing of children (Spencer 1994a: 328), but only if there is 'evidence of abuse' and avoiding an 'infringement of privacy', which conveniently ignores the fact that these are incompatible goals. Yet such intrusions are an inevitable consequence of any policy that defines some people as 'illegal', or in Spencer's euphemism, 'irregular'.

I make these points about *Strangers and Citizens* to demonstrate the problems entailed in the advancement of 'fair' immigration controls. Even if one does not accept that controls are racist and discriminatory at their core, the effects of attempting to implement them are contradictory and discriminatory, whatever convolutions advocates may use to make them otherwise.

Stonewall, an organisation which campaigns for the rights of gay men and lesbians, has contributed to the debate on immigration controls, as a result of discrimination against same-sex partners wishing to live together in the UK (Stonewall Immigration Group 2000). Their demand has been for equal treatment with other family units. This is based on an assumption that immigration controls are necessary, but as they stand, privilege recognised heterosexual families. In fact all heterosexual families are not treated equally under immigration policies. There is a pattern of differential treatment of families seeking entry into the UK from Asia and Africa, and those from countries such as Australia, Canada and USA (rich, largely white countries).

Stonewall's demands have to some extent been met, in that from 2 October 2000, the Immigration Rules permit entry to same-sex partners who have lived together for at least two of the preceding three years, as is the case for heterosexuals. However the discrimination continues in that there is a requirement for a further two years together to obtain permanent settlement (one year for married heterosexuals). Even if further concessions are made, lesbian and gay partnerships would still be subject to the racism that underpins the legislation. The question remains, which 'families' do Stonewall want to be equal with? As Cohen says, calling for non-discriminatory immigration controls 'makes as much sense as arguing for equal opportunities for black people in apartheid' (Cohen 1995: 22).

The case against immigration controls

First, the position taken in this chapter is an opposition to all immigration controls in principle, on the grounds that the very notion of creating external controls on people's right to enter a country, and internal controls on their movements and entitlement to the country's resources, depend on nationalist and racist assumptions and cannot under any circumstances be justified. The discussion in this section starts from that assumption.

As noted earlier, a variety of writers and groups argue against immigration controls. However in some cases the grounds on which they do this are suspect, and the rationale that underpins their position is susceptible to being appropriated to favour imposing controls and is therefore a hostage to fortune. Here I consider some of these arguments, both from those on the political Left, and from those on the libertarian Right.

The political Left

The arguments from the Left against immigration controls depend on rules of debate that are based on binary opposites, similar to those employed by advocates of 'just' and 'unjust', 'fair' and 'unfair' actions of government. The pamphlet published by the Socialist Workers Party, *The Case Against Immigration Controls* (Taylor nd), illustrates the problems. Taylor sets out the 'facts' as follows.

There are more people entering Britain than leaving. The figures set out by Taylor (nd: 6) are useful in demonstrating the pattern of movement, and in confirming the racist nature of restrictions against people from Africa and Asia, but it is not helpful to support the argument against immigration controls by concluding that the recent figures show more leaving than entering. What if the figures were to show that more immigrants and others were entering than leaving (and official statistics are notoriously malleable – see Levitas and Guy 1996)? Moreover, one can envisage that even where figures are used in this way to argue against immigration controls, there will be voices raised to point to the hoards of 'illegal' immigrants, who do not appear in official statistics. The argument is easily turned to become one that supports controls. In any case it seems rather naïve of Taylor to take official statistics at face value.

Immigrants and refugees are almost exclusively young (Taylor nd: 7). The rationale here is that Britain has an ageing population, with increasing proportions of the population over age 65, and people over 80 living longer. As part of the working population, the argument goes, young people arriving here make contributions towards pensions and health care, thus helping to solve the problem of an ageing population and of people in paid work. Taylor would be interested to know that this is an argument also being used currently by the New Labour Government to cope with a perceived skills shortage (Roche 2000). It has also been used by Findlay (in Spencer 1994a) to argue for 'fair' immigration controls. This could easily become a justification for excluding older people from entry to the UK. And what is the definition of 'young', since this varies, and large numbers of workers are being made redundant in their forties and fifties (Novak 1996)? And when the demographic trends in Britain shift towards a younger population, it is easy (given the history of controls), to forecast arguments that 'they are taking our jobs'. In such a situation, is it likely that old people will be admitted and young people excluded, since old people do not threaten jobs? Moreover, young immigrants grow old eventually, and will need pensions themselves. This argument about the contribution young people could make to the economy also ignores the social context, where cultural stereotypes of young black men in particular, view them as not productive, as criminal and as dangerous, and therefore as 'undesirable'. The question arises as to *which* young people are to be welcomed.

Taylor's arguments implicitly draw on a rationale underpinned by the needs of the economy, a very precarious foundation on which to build an argument for ending immigration controls, since the needs of the economy will change. Britain is a good example of this in its government's attempts to attract workers from the Caribbean in the 1950s, only to be followed by the introduction of stringent controls on entry in the 1960s, reinforced by the promotion of images of bloody racial strife without controls. That the politician, Enoch Powell (Health Minister in the 1950s), was centrally involved in both of these strategies, is a vivid illustration of the ways 'rational' arguments against immigration controls can be co-opted to support the binary opposite as expedience demands. When Immigration Minister, Barbara Roche (in a speech sponsored by the British Bankers Association), states that Britain now needs to attract workers from abroad who will enhance the economy, she has in mind 'the brightest and best talents – the entrepreneurs, the scientists, the high technology specialists who make the global economy tick' (Roche 2000: 1).

This need to attract workers is one that preoccupies other EU countries, as well as the USA. Both Britain and the USA have sent delegations to India to attract techno-migrants with all the skills of the new technology. In the USA a fee of $1000 will be charged to employers for each visa issued, raising an estimated $170 million earmarked for training Americans seeking these skills. Immigrants who apply for visas without specific technical skills, will not be considered. Visas issued will be on a *temporary* basis (*Guardian*, 30 October 2000). Alongside this, it is estimated that around 12 per cent of the workforce is made up of 'illegal' immigrants working in sweatshops, as farm workers and in service industries. Some of the big trade unions have dropped their opposition to illegal, undocumented labour, since many occupations now depend on workers who have no choice but to accept low wages and poor conditions. In the UK, apart from questions about what 'poaching' Indian workers will do to India, one might ask whether the qualifications of technicians will have equal recognition with those gained in the UK, whether the deal will include permanent settlement, and if not, what will happen to the workers when their contract ends.

Roche's speech included a revealing contradiction, which underlines the intention that only skilled workers will be sought. She referred to the 1905 Aliens Act and to the anti-Semitic comment from an MP at the time, that it is 'the poorest and least fit of these people who move', identifying herself as their descendent, having achieved the high office of Immigration Minister. The message here is that immigrants (even the poor and the sick) potentially enhance and enrich the British culture. Yet her speech went on to attack 'bogus' asylum seekers and those without a 'well-founded claim' – in other words, similar arguments to those that were used to keep out Jewish people at the turn of the nineteenth century. Who then is the arbiter of what is a 'good' contribution, and who is to decide what would be a 'bad' effect on the country? We have seen that the 'needs of the labour market' is a position argued for by the political Left to support 'no immigration controls'. We have also seen it turned on its head by conservative forces supporting controls on the very same grounds – 'in the national interest'. Although British governments have not ruled out asylum on humanitarian grounds, arguments about the needs of the economy tend to override other concerns, and indeed are used to exclude those whose motives are constructed as being 'economic' rather than humanitarian.

The SWP pamphlet by Taylor (nd) sets out other dimensions of their case against immigration controls – there are not too few jobs, refugees are not scroungers dependent on 'welfare', there is enough housing for all. All of these can be interrogated on the same terms as I have set out above, and will collapse when challenged, because of their flawed logic. I hope the point has been made that the tactic of many of those who oppose immigration controls, to enter into the debate on the same terms of those who advocate immigration controls, is naïve and susceptible to appropriation as social conditions change or are differently constructed.

The libertarian Right

Another source for arguments against immigration controls comes from the libertarian Right. The basic premise of libertarianism is that individuals have the right to live in any way they choose so long as they respect the equal rights of others. The only actions to be forbidden by law are those that involve the initiation of force. Libertarians oppose government actions such as censorship, price controls, confiscation of property and regulation of people's personal and economic lives. The Cato Institute, a USA-based, libertarian organisation that argues for limited government, free markets and individual liberty, includes in its policies an opposition to immigration controls. Along with the National Immigration Forum, it published a report entitled *Immigration: the demographic and economic facts* (Cato Institute 1995), supported by 40 other groups including Asian, Caribbean, Jewish, Christian, human rights, refugee and lawyers' organisations in the USA. The report rehearsed similar arguments to those of Taylor about the quantities of immigrants, their economic contribution, taxes paid, education, their use of welfare, their impact on natural resources, and so on. The overall conclusion was that *both legal and illegal* immigrants make a rich contribution to the life of the nation. This sentiment has recently been incorporated into a briefing document for Congress (Cato Institute 2000). However this document is revealing in that it appears to accept the categories 'legal' and 'illegal', by recommending that the issues of legal and illegal immigration should be kept separate (Cato Institute 2000: 8). Significantly, it also recommends *deregulating employment-based immigration*, 'the current regulatory scheme bears no relation to the competitive way companies recruit in the real world and should be eliminated or reformed to reflect market forces' (Cato Institute 2000: 8). In other words, it is companies' and employers' liberty that is being protected here, and immigrants are being placed in the role of commodity. The fact that the Cato Institute also opposes measures that would protect workers' rights – proper wage legislation, conducive job conditions, health and safety obligations, strong unions, and so on – all necessary to prevent exploitation, reinforces this conclusion. The notion of individual freedoms advantages those who are already economically powerful, and it is in their interests that the Cato Institute operates. As for would-be immigrants, those who have resources and the choice to move at will, might benefit. Indeed they will be the people and institutions least likely to be subject to controls in the present regime. Many people are not able to move easily, nor would they *choose* to leave their country of origin. In the modern world immigration patterns are characterised largely by *compulsion*, not choice. Real freedom would not result in people being compelled to migrate thousands of miles from the place they regard as home. The libertarian position encourages the exploitation of vulnerable groups and advantages the powerful and affluent.

Nationalism and racism at the heart of immigration controls

The argument put forward here against immigration controls, is simply and solely that they are fundamentally and irretrievably based on nationalist and racist sentiments. In my use of 'nationalism' it is important to distinguish between those nationalisms that constitute a struggle against colonial and imperial domination towards the liberation of downtrodden peoples, and those hegemonic nationalisms that involve themselves as authors of that very oppression, resulting in extreme cases, in 'ethnic cleansing' and extermination. Here I am concerned with the link between nationalism and racism, and examine briefly the ideas that underpin nationalism, and their racist connection to immigration policies. For discussion of nationalism and racism in more depth, see Anderson (1983), Anthias and Yuval-Davis (1989), Goldberg (1993), Miles (1993), Yuval-Davis (1997) and Cohen (2001).

The issue is that underpinning all immigration controls are notions of nationalism and chauvinism. All immigration laws depend on the distinction between 'native' and 'foreigner', 'citizen' and 'alien', 'us' and 'them', and therefore 'legal' and 'illegal'. Each of these polarities depends on its opposite for it to have any meaning at all. 'Legal' has no meaning unless we can identify 'illegal'. And supporting these binaries are the other, racially marked binaries: civilised/uncivilised, cultured/primitive, monogamous/polygamous, rational/emotional, and so on. The setting up of boundaries involves the management of identities and cultures in inclusionary and exclusionary ways. Where these boundaries are related to concepts of 'nation', there are a number of features that make up the myth of the national character, which construct it both as 'natural' and familiar. The opposite of the national character is simultaneously constructed as undesirable and foreign, thus justifying exclusion. What are some of the ingredients of this nationalism?

The homogeneous national 'character' and identity

First, nationalism depends on a myth of homogeneity amongst the people, what Smith calls a 'myth–symbol complex' (Smith 1986: 18) and Anderson calls an 'imagined community . . . not the awakening of nations to self-consciousness: it *invents* nations where they do not exist' (Anderson 1983: 6). Nations are not 'natural' communities, arising from a common stock or kinship. The 'nation' is a creation, and nationalism the ideology drawn upon to legitimate the actions of the state. Teresa Hayter (2000) describes in detail the variety of origins of the people of the British Isles, demonstrating that Britain is the product of generations of immigrants. The following poem captures the process:

> *The Paleolithic, Stone and Bronze Age races*
> *The Celt, the Roman, Teutons not a few*
> *Diverse in dialects and hair and faces –*
> *The Fleming, Dutchman, Huguenot and Jew*
> *'Tis hard to prove by means authoritative*
> *Which is the alien and which the native.*
>
> (Quoted by Cohen 1994)

Yet in spite of Britain, like most countries, being the product of immigration, notions of national culture and nationality homogeneity still have potency. This homogeneity includes images of shared origins and destiny, a shared culture and customs, values and religion, and significantly, shared *blood*. In this way 'race' is insinuated in a common breeding population. Any differences or inequalities are subsumed in a sense of belonging to a national family, often symbolised by a royal family, or as in the USA by a 'first' family, or a female figure as 'mother of the nation' (such as 'Britannia'). The nation is always conceived as a 'deep, horizontal comradeship' (Anderson 1983: 7), invoking a patriotism for which people will die if called upon to do so. The language of 'common descent' gives constructed social relations a veneer of fixedness. As Goldberg (1993: 80) comments, 'group formation seems destined as eternal, fated as unchanging and unchangeable'. As a result, people who have nothing in common, who have nothing to do with each other, and indeed whose interests are objectively in conflict, are brought together in a common self-perception. From a position inside this myth, the foreigner, the outsider, the alien, the Other, can be constructed.

The process of Othering

The notion of the national character for the purposes of immigration controls, requires not only an inclusive identity for those defined as 'of the national family', but also the other end of the binary, the process of

Othering, the construction of the outsider, the foreigner, the unwashed, the candidate for exclusion. It serves to create myths that have boundaries that are both exclusive and inclusive. The concept of 'race' helps to define the parameters of 'nation', and racism is at the heart of the construction of the Other. A number of writers have offered theories of Othering (for example de Beauvoir 1949/53; Fanon 1970, Lacan 1977, Said 1978). Key to these approaches is the idea that particular groups are represented as Others in ways which reinforce the power and purported superiority of those with control over the processes of representation. Historically, those constituted as Other include subject peoples within global structures of material exploitation, but there are multiple fissures across lines of 'race', class, gender, sexual identity, disability and age for example, which are drawn upon in different contexts to reinforce the 'difference' of those to be excluded. All of the dimensions mentioned here have at one time or another and in a variety of ways, been drawn into justifications for immigration controls.

In terms of 'race', McClintock shows the ways in which the concept has been used in unstable and shifting ways, 'sometimes as synonymous with "species", sometimes with "culture", sometimes with "nation", sometimes to denote biological ethnicity or sub-groups within national groupings: the English "race" compared say, with the "Irish" race' (McClintock 1995: 52). At the end of the nineteenth century members of the Ethnological Society were able to establish an 'Index of Nigrescence', for the peoples of Britain and Ireland. Irish people were labelled 'white negroes', 'Irish Iberians' and 'Celtic Calibans' to locate them low in the racial hierarchy, but manifestly above people of African origin.

Although these images no longer have credibility in their crude form, they illustrate the processes of racialisation – the identification of any group as having characteristics that construct them as an inferior and often dangerous 'race', not fit for inclusion in the national family, and worthy only of the most menial of work outside the borders of society, or of exclusion altogether. Such ideas are the modern subtext of ethnic cleansing and genocide. They are also at the heart of treatment of Muslims and Roma people who arrived in the UK seeking asylum from oppression in countries of Eastern Europe. The assumptions that underpin these ideas continue to justify not only exclusion, but discrimination, poor treatment and violence against minorities within countries.

In any country where the rights to enter and to remain are policed, decisions have to be made as to who 'belongs' and who does not, who is 'legal' and who is 'illegal'. The path for this has to be prepared in the ways described above. And the grounds on which these judgements are made are *ideological*. As Yuval-Davis says:

The 'freedom of movement within the European Community', the Israeli Law of Return and the patriality clause in British immigration legislation – all are instances of ideological, often racist, constructions of boundaries which allow unrestricted immigration to some and block it completely to others.

(Yuval-Davis 1997: 74)

The justification for border controls depends on the persuasiveness of these inclusionary and exclusionary nationalist and racially informed arguments. In this sense, the existence of policies in favour of immigration control is intrinsically dependent on the acceptance of the assumptions that underpin them. It is clear then, that there cannot be 'fair', non-racist immigration controls.

The dominant discourses within immigration control

The construction of the undesirable Other, described above, has been central to the tactics used to 'soften up' public opinion in preparation for the introduction of legislation, since the dawn of immigration controls (see Chapter 3 of this volume for an historical overview; also Cohen 1996). Images of Jewish communities as 'a seething mass of refuse and filth' (Garrard 1971: 51), and of diseased and poor stock, fed fears about the contamination of British blood and the weakening of the British lineage. At the same time – the other side of the binary – there was seen to be a need to breed an Imperial race in Great Britain (Semmell 1960), to retain a strong Empire. The construction of the British welfare state was explicitly a provision for strengthening those seen to belong to Nation (Chapter 3 of this volume; Cohen 1996). In the 1950s the themes of inclusion and exclusion were rehearsed in connection with black immigration. In their contemporary form they employ the language of 'our people', 'our services', against 'bogus', 'parasite', 'economic migrants', fuelling spectres of welfare scroungers and job thieves (Harding 2000).

The 1962 Commonwealth Immigrants Act, which introduced the concept of 'patriality', set the parameters of claims to British nationality. 'Patriality' was incorporated in the 1981 Nationality Act, as a result of which five different 'British' nationalities were created, only one of which allowed free access to the country. Thus people labelled 'British Overseas Citizen', 'Citizen of Dependent Territories', 'British Subject', 'Hong Kong Citizen' were not afforded right of entry. This was reserved for those with a 'real' British nationality – 'British Citizens'. What was written into the legislation was the myth of a distinct race of people of common origin and descent: white and European. Henceforth, British nationality could be claimed only by those with a grandparent born in Britain, a provision that effectively excluded swathes of people from the Asian subcontinent and the Caribbean. As a result of this, between 1981 and 1983, refusal rates for applications for family reunion of people from the Indian subcontinent rose from 30 per cent to 44 per cent (Spencer 1997). White South Africans and white Zimbabweans could gain entry, but not black citizens of these countries. This is a classic example of the coming together of nationalism and racism to exclude the unwelcome Other. Immigration laws cannot be sanitised, or made non-racist. They are inherently racist.

The dynamic nature of racist policies

Not only are immigration controls racist in their treatment of people wishing to enter the country, their effect connects with and feeds perceptions of particular groups *within* the country, which constructs them as outsiders and legitimates discrimination against them in a host of ways. In Britain, ever since the Aliens Act of 1905, immigration controls have linked external control of borders with internal control of access to political rights, employment, welfare benefits and social services (Cohen 1996; 2001). Those perceived as 'different', regardless of immigration status, are increasingly required to prove their entitlement to services. They are regarded as not 'of' the nation.

Although the biggest impact of this is on British people who are visibly 'different', to argue that black people are the only groups affected would be to condemn black communities to being perpetual victims and to deny the changing manifestations of racism. The history of immigration controls teaches us that although the underlying racist character of such controls is unchanging, the groups who are identified as Other and as Alien may change over time. The *dynamic* nature of racism is such that at different times we have seen Jews, Irish people, Asians, Africans and African–Caribbean people excluded or subject to internal controls. There is of course a thread of continuity of discrimination against these groups which is still apparent and which is embodied in legislation. And the character of racism still discriminates between white and black. However the contemporary manifestation of the racist phenomenon also encompasses Bosnians, Kosovans and others displaced from Eastern Europe. To essentialise and fix the character of racism, a mistake of some commentators on the Left (which incidentally mirrors the fixity of the myth of the national character, so beloved of the Right), is to be out of touch with its many guises, and to be running to catch up with its nasty trail of destruction.

Conclusion

It is true, for the reasons given by Hayter (2000), that immigration controls simply do not work, and they result in human misery and suffering. However, the position taken here against controls is that there is one argument for anti-racists, which is not at risk of appropriation by those who argue in favour of controls. There can never be immigration controls that are not institutionally racist, and therefore there can be no defensible justification of them:

> It is time for the idea of international migration to be rescued, and enshrined in international declarations as a normal and a natural right. It is time also to question the assumption that governments and their citizens have the right to exercise control in their own interest over particular bits of land, any more than they have the right to appropriate the air and the sea.
>
> (Hayter 2000: 151)

The Macpherson Report (1999) on the death of Stephen Lawrence held that the British police service is 'institutionally racist'. This has been interpreted to mean different things to different groups. However it is defined, it might be argued that the police service and other state institutions need not be *inevitably* institutionally racist. One could envisage a non-racist police force and a non-racist welfare state. Immigration legislation can never be envisaged as racism-free. It and the apparatus that supports it, are uniquely intrinsically racist.

This is not to say that I see the abolition of immigration controls as a panacea for all ills, or as the only action that needs to be taken. There remain a number of thorny questions. If there were a world of free movement, for example, migrant labour would still need to be protected from profit-seeking private capital, and humanitarian principles would still have to be observed. Countries such as Cuba would still need protection from *saboteurs*, and other (particularly third world) countries from the arrival of capital seeking cheap labour.

There is also the issue of whether, as some political placards have it, 'All immigrants are welcome here' and 'Hands off my friend' (*Socialist Worker*, 11 November 2000), is a defensible position. Does the 'welcome' include international criminals such as General Pinochet, the Iranian Secret Police and others who have committed genocide and other atrocities and are fleeing from justice in their own countries? Does it include people such as Mike Tyson, convicted of rape in the USA, but supported by many black people as the victim of a racist

218   *Beth Humphries*

jury? One of the problems in this notion of active *welcome*, this 'christianisation' of opposition to immigration controls, is that not all of us would actively welcome those whose political or religious views we find objectionable and oppressive, but whose right to asylum we would uphold if they are fleeing from persecution. We do not need to see those subject to immigration controls as our 'friends', or to have them on our side politically. This of course begs the question, if the state were to outlaw fascists, would we be obliged to demand their entry? At the same time, who is to arbitrate on what is 'crime' and what is say, 'liberation struggle'? The actions of hegemonic, racist and imperialist states signal caution about an uncritical acceptance of definitions of criminality as unproblematic.

There is also the related issue of internal exile, possible in Britain through anti-terrorism legislation, as a result of which people in mainland Britain may be exiled to the North of Ireland and refused further entry to Britain. Is this a material recognition that the Irish – northern or southern, are 'with' us, but still not 'of' us?

These and many other questions remain. I am aware that a policy of 'no immigration controls' will be regarded as an impractical and impossible dream. It is salutary to remember that the introduction of controls is a recent, twentieth-century phenomenon. To have no immigration controls is not the salvation of humanity, but it is a beginning, and it would be a major structural shift, signalling a genuine commitment to an anti-racist world.

References

Anderson, B. (1983) *Imagined Communities,* London: Verso.
Anthias, F. and Yuval-Davis, N. (1989) *Woman–Nation–State,* London: Macmillan.
Carens, J. H. (1987) 'Aliens and Citizens: the case for open borders', *Review of Politics,* 49(2): 251–273.
Cato Institute (1995) *Immigration: the demographic and economic facts,* Washington DC: Cato Institute and the National Immigration Forum. http://www.cato.org/pubs/policy_report/pr-immih.html.
—— (2000) *Cato Handbook for Congress. No.29. Immigration,* Washington DC: Cato Institute. http://www.cato.org//pubs/handbook/hb105–29.html.
Cohen, R. (1994) *Frontiers of Identity: the British and the Others,* London: Longman.
Cohen, S. (1995) *Workers' Control, Not Immigration Controls,* Manchester: Greater Manchester Immigration Unit.
—— (1996) 'Anti-semitism, immigration controls and the welfare state', in D. Taylor (ed.) *Critical Social Policy: a reader,* London: Sage, pp 24–47.

—— (2001) *Immigration Controls, the Family and the Welfare State*, London: Jessica Kingsley Publishers.

de Beauvoir, S. (1949/53) *The Second Sex*, New York: Knopf.

Dummett, A. and Nicol, A. (1990) *Subjects, Citizens, Aliens and Others*, London: Weidenfeld and Nicolson.

Fanon, F. (1970) *Black Skin, White Masks*, London: Paladin.

Garrard, J. A. (1971) *The English and Immigration: a comparative study of the Jewish influx, 1880–1910*, London: Oxford University Press.

Goldberg, D. T. (1993) *Racist Culture*, Oxford: Blackwell.

Harding, J. (2000) *The Uninvited: refugees at the rich man's gate*, London: Profile.

Harnisch, A., Stokes, A.M. and Wedauer, F. (eds) (1998*) Fringe Voices*, Oxford and New York: Berg.

Hayter, T. (2000) *Open Borders: the case against immigration controls*, London: Pluto Press.

Lacan, J. (1977) *Ecrits: a selection*, London: Routledge.

Levitas, R. and Guy, W. (1996) *Interpreting Official Statistics*, London: Routledge.

McClintock, A. (1995) *Imperial Leather: race, gender and sexuality in the colonial context*, New York: Routledge.

Macpherson Report (1999) *The Stephen Lawrence Inquiry: report of an inquiry by Sir William Macpherson of Cluny* (M4262–1/2), London: The Stationery Office.

Miles, R. (1993) *Racism after 'Race Relations'*, London: Routledge.

Novak (1996) 'Empowerment and the politics of poverty', in B. Humphries (ed.) *Critical Perspectives on Empowerment*, Birmingham: Venture Press, pp 85–98.

Roche, B. (2000) 'UK migration in a global economy', Speech given at a seminar organised by the Institute of Public Relations Policy and British Bankers Association.

Said, E. (1978) *Orientalism*, London: Routledge & Kegan Paul.

Semmell, B. (1960) *Imperialism and Social Reform: English social-imperial thought 1895–1914*, London: Allen & Unwin.

Smith, A. D. (1986) *The Ethnic Origin of Nations*, Oxford: Basil Blackwell.

Spencer, I. R. G. (1997) *British Immigration Policy since 1939: the making of multi-racial Britain*, London: Routledge.

Spencer, S. (ed.) (1994a) *Strangers and Citizens: a positive approach to migrants and refugees*, London: Rivers Oram Press.

Spencer, S. (ed.) (1994b) *Immigration as an Economic Asset: the German experience*, Stoke-on-Trent: IPPR/Trentham Books.

Stonewall Immigration Group (2000) *Briefing Document on Immigration Rules*. http: //www.stonewall-immigration.org.uk/The%20Concession.htm.

Yuval-Davis, N. (1997) *Gender and Nation*, London: Sage.

Zimmerman, K. F. (1994) 'The labour market impact of immigration', in S. Spencer (ed), *Immigration as an Economic Asset: the German experience*, Stoke-on-Trent: IPPR/Trentham Books, pp 39–64.

13 In and against the state of immigration controls

Strategies for resistance

Steve Cohen

Introduction

Asylum seekers calling for an immediate end to the controversial voucher scheme brought chaos to a supermarket [Kwik Save in Hull] yesterday with a blockade which shut tills all afternoon.

(*Guardian*, 2 October 2000)

For the last three months asylum seekers housed in the hostel [Rose Lodge Court, Langley Green, West Midlands] have been complaining about conditions in the hostel – cramped living conditions, stodgy food and inadequate health care. There have been several hunger strikes and this week things came to a head with a roof top protest, occupation of the main road and a sit-in hunger strike . . . twenty of the asylum seekers, mostly Iraqi and Iranian Kurds are now planning to march to NASS headquarters in Croydon.

(Press release, National Coalition of
Anti-Deportation Campaigns, 8 September 2000)

Iranian asylum-seekers in Newcastle went on hunger strike after being housed alongside political enemies from Iraq and having their financial support cut. They claimed they were being treated like prisoners.

(*Newcastle Evening Chronicle*, 29 May 2000)

On Monday 25 September, at 11pm, armed German border police raided asylum camp number 5 in the city of Zwickau, South-East Germany, in order to arrest and deport two Lebanese families. . . . A struggle ensued between the police and around 300 asylum seekers. At 3.30 am the police were forced to retreat without the two families.

(Press release, International Federation of
Iranian Refugees, 27 September 2000)

The issues

There has been resistance to controls from when they were first proposed in the nineteenth century. The examples at the start of this
chapter are simply the latest manifestations of this resistance, both in
the UK and elsewhere. However, they are significant examples in that
they show struggles taking place not directly over the demand to come
or stay here. These struggles are taking place on issues of welfare, or
more accurately they are occurring where welfare control meets immigration control. The whole development over the last century has been
a growing synthesis between welfare entitlements and immigration
status. This has achieved a qualitative leap with the 1999 Immigration
and Asylum Act. This Act has created a new poor law for asylum seekers based on a cashless voucher economy and accommodation
provision via forced dispersal.

The above examples are showing resistance, collective resistance, by
those subject to welfare control based on immigration status. In essence,
this is resistance against the state. However, this chapter is also concerned with another group. This group comprises workers employed
within national and local welfare agencies who now find that they have
become agents of the Home Office and of internal immigration controls. They have been given the role of investigators of immigration
status in order to determine entitlement to benefits or services.
Examples of welfare provision, linked, though not necessarily in the
same ways, to status are: housing under both the homelessness provisions and allocation from the housing register; further and higher
education fees and loans; in-patient hospital treatment; housing benefit;
council tax benefit; other basic means-tested benefits; non-contributory
sickness and disability benefits; child benefit; support under community
care provisions contained within Section 21 of the 1948 National
Assistance Act (adult residential care); Section 45 of the 1968 Health
Services and Public Health Act (services for frail elderly people) and
Schedule 8 of the 1977 National Health Services Act (day care services
for the ill); support for children and families under Section 17 of the
1989 Children Act.[1]

The legislation linking status to entitlement places in a collusive position workers within the health service, those employed by the Benefits
Agency, finance officers within tertiary education and a whole range of
local authority workers. This poses the question of what struggles, if
any, have been waged against their collusive role by this group. *In and
Against The State* (London to Edinburgh Weekend Return Group 1979)
was a seminal agitational work, calling for an alliance between users of

welfare and workers within welfare – an alliance in defence of welfare. Significantly this did not refer to the unholy nexus between immigration status and welfare entitlement, though admittedly this was far less visible than now. This chapter bases itself on this earlier pioneering study, and extends it into the relationships of immigration controls and welfare. Within these relationships it looks at struggles from without and sabotage from within.

This chapter is about ideas and action, ideology and resistance. It is in support of an ideology that is against all immigration controls. It is opposed to all ideologies that argue for the possibility of 'fair' controls. It is in support of resistance to all controls by whatever means. As such it addresses an issue relevant to struggles both in and against the state. A central question in all political endeavour is the relationship between ideas and action. In what way has the latter been determined by the former, or in what way could it be determined? Is there always a one-to-one relationship between the two or is this crude reductionism? Within the context of immigration controls and of welfare entitlements based on such controls the question is posed as to whether it makes any difference whatsoever whether resistance is posed in terms of opposition to all controls or in terms of a demand that controls be rendered 'fair'. This therefore requires an examination of these two distinct ideological positions, a task undertaken by Humphries in Chapter 12 of this volume.

The two camps

Support for a position of no immigration restrictions is a minority position, even amongst those critical of controls. The dominant ideological position is that which argues for 'fair' or 'reasonable' or 'just' controls. The most lengthy exposition of this view can be found in the collection of essays *Strangers and Citizens*, edited by Sarah Spencer (1994). This is co-published by the Institute of Public Policy Research. The IPPR is closely allied to the Labour Party. Immigration Ministers sometimes use the IPPR as a platform to launch policy statements. Barbara Roche announced her elitist proposal to encourage 'quality' immigration at an IPPR conference (12 September 2000; see also Cohen 2000). Indeed Roche's ideas were closely modelled on proposals in *Strangers and Citizens* and in particular on proposals within Allan Findlay's essay, 'An economic audit of contemporary immigration' (in Spencer 1994). In fact, the main organisational proponent of 'fair' controls is the trade union and labour movement. The clearest example of this is seen in the Report of the 1990 Trades Union Congress. Ron

Todd spoke on behalf of the TUC General Council asking that a resolution by NALGO be remitted as it implied opposition to all controls.[2]
It was remitted. Ron Todd is quoted in the Report as saying 'We support the Labour Party's plans to replace the 1971, 1981[3] and 1988
Immigration Acts with rules and practices which no longer discriminate
on the grounds of race and sex. But we have to be clear that this is not
the same as outright repeal' (see Cohen 1995: 22).

The literature of those arguing for outright repeal is extraordinarily
small (but see Cohen 1995; 2001; Hayter 2000). On the other hand
there is a major movement for the abolition of all controls – though it
is not a movement which necessarily always or openly articulates this
demand. What is being referred to here are campaigns against deportation. These operate as flying pickets against immigration laws.
Campaigns against deportation in essence deny state authority to
impose controls. Indeed the emphasis, particularly within the Labour
Party and therefore Labour Government, on the need for 'fair' controls
is itself a response to the culture of resistance against deportations.
Prior to this culture emerging in the 1970s there was no discourse in
favour of fair controls. The call for 'fair' laws was a successful political
attempt to reassert authority by the state to impose controls, in language designed to make controls appear acceptable.

History of resistance pre-1945

Resistance to controls is as old as controls themselves (see Cohen 1996).
Indeed, it predates the enactment of controls. The first UK immigration
laws were contained in the 1905 Aliens Act. This was directed against
Jewish refugees fleeing anti-Semitism in Eastern Europe and Tsarist
Russia. Jewish workers organised, though without success, against the
proposed legislation. The *Jewish Chronicle* of 21 August 1894 reported
a rally in London's Whitechapel area, against the support of the TUC
for controls. A resolution was passed declaring that 'This mass meeting
of Jewish trade unionists is of the opinion that the vast amount of
poverty and misery which exists is in no way due to the influx of foreign
workmen, but is the result of the private ownership of the means of
production and this meeting calls upon the government to pass a universal compulsory eight hours day with a minimum wage as an
instalment of future reform'. In 1895 ten, mainly Jewish, trade unions,
produced a pamphlet against controls titled *A voice from the Aliens*.
This was launched at rallies held in London and Leeds, with the
London meeting being addressed by Eleanor Marx and the Russian
anarchist Prince Kropotkin (*Jewish Chronicle*, 13 August 1895). The

Jewish Chronicle of 24 January 1902 reported the establishment of an Aliens Defence League, based in Brick Lane, to fight controls. In September 1902 there was a major indoor rally against the proposed legislation at the Wonderland in Whitechapel. The *Eastern Post and City Chronicle* of 20 September reported that 'the hall, capable of accommodating three thousand people was filled to its utmost capacity and still thousands clamoured for admission'.

All this activity represented a peak of resistance to controls for another six decades. After the defeat of the opposition to the controls embodied in the Aliens Act, resistance was not organised or collective, nor did it take to the streets. Instead, the opposition took the form of literary opposition and lobbying of ministers. For instance the operation of the Aliens Act was subjected to trenchant criticism by the *Jewish Chronicle*. Between 1906 and 1914[4] the paper reported weekly on refusals of entry and appeals against these refusals. In 1907 (11 October–5 November) it ran a series of articles on *The Aliens Act and its Administration*. The sub-heading to the first article described the Act as 'an un-English piece of legislation, saturated with class prejudice from almost the first clause to the last and divorced from every true democratic instinct. It has proved itself arbitrary, retrograde, tyrannical and cruel'. The description 'an un-English piece of legislation' was misconceived and just the opposite of reality. What the Aliens Act politically achieved (and subsequent legislation politically strengthened) was to provide a definition of the state in terms of who was allowed entry into the territory and who was allowed to remain there. Other than this, the *Jewish Chronicle* provided a description of immigration control which could also apply to all subsequent immigration restrictions. In 1911, M.J. Landa's book, *The Alien Problem and Its Remedy* was published, attacking the Act.

Parallel to this literary opposition was the occasional lobbying of ministers by what was, in essence, the Jewish elite. This lobbying took the form of either personal deputations or correspondence. For instance, the *Jewish Chronicle* of 10 June 1910 reported a letter from Winston Churchill, then Home Secretary, to the Board of Deputies of British Jewry. This followed two requests by the Board. One was for the provision of 'receiving houses' near the docks where immigrant ships landed, so that those appealing refusal of entry could stay there whilst awaiting their appeal (otherwise they were constrained to remain on board ship). The second request was for appellants to have the right to legal representation in the appeal. Churchill agreed with the first demand, but not the second.

Resistance against controls and for the entry of refugees did not reach the pre-1905 level, even at the time of the Nazification of Germany, Austria and Czechoslovakia. Though there was much criticism of the UK's refusal to open its borders, this again seems to have been confined to literary criticisms and deputations to ministers (see London 1999).[5] This contrasts with the active political opposition to fascism in Spain and its home-grown variant in this country.

History of resistance post-1945

Opposition to controls post-1945 has been militant and collective, and has taken place at grassroots level. It has reflected the growing political strength of the black community, and has operated as a barometer of that strength. The 1962 Commonwealth Immigrants Act was the first post-war legislation. It was aimed at the entry of black commonwealth citizens. The *West Indian Gazette*, edited by Claudia Jones,[6] campaigned consistently against the proposed Act, with one entire issue, that of December 1961, being devoted to this. The *Daily Worker* of 10 November 1961 reported on the publication of a pamphlet against the legislation produced jointly by the Indian Workers Association, the Pakistani Workers Association and the West Indian Workers Association. This was entitled *Immigration – can control be justified?* The *Daily Worker* also reported on various, relatively small, activities against the proposed law, including for instance a midnight picket of the Home Office consisting of 'several hundred' people (12 February 1962). Activities against the 1968 Commonwealth Immigrants Act and the 1971 Immigration Act were progressively bigger. The *Morning Star* (the *Daily Worker*'s successor) reported a demonstration of 'more than 3000 people' to Downing Street against the 1968 legislation. The *Guardian* of 22 March 1971 reported a march of 'about 5000' people to Whitehall protesting the 1971 Bill.

Protests against every piece of subsequent legislation have grown in size. However, the defining and historically unique feature of the last quarter of a century has been resistance to the deportation of black individuals and families. The first such campaigns appear to be that of Saeed Rahman in 1977 and Abdul Azad in 1978 in Bradford.[7] Anti-deportation campaigns have been significant in many ways. First they have been rooted in the black community. Second, they have thrown up their own leadership and have not been based on self-appointed 'community leaders'. Third, they have relied on neither Parliament nor the courts to succeed, but on their own strength. Fourth, they refuse to go away. Indeed, during the Thatcher years they probably represented the most consistent form of extra-parliamentary opposition to government generally and the Home Office in particular.

Fifth, this consistent, on-going and exemplary activity by black people has legitimised post-1945 resistance to controls. As such it has facilitated the development within the last decade of resistance by asylum seekers. This last point is important as the modern movement of asylum seekers rarely acknowledges its roots in the movement of black people against controls, just as this latter resistance rarely acknowledged its heritage in the self-activity of Jewish refugees in the first half of the twentieth century. Historical memory has a short lifespan when it comes to opposition to immigration controls.

In and against the state

All the above examples of opposition were against the state. However, they were not from 'within' any of its agencies and particularly its welfare agencies. This poses the following questions. First, what opposition has there been to the increasing nexus between welfare entitlement and immigration status? Second, how much of this opposition has come from within welfare? Third, what form has been taken by any opposition – has it gone beyond commentary, criticism and propaganda and assumed a more active role? Opposition can itself be a continuum, ranging from verbal or literary observation to full-blooded revolution.

Modern welfare legislation at its very inception linked entitlement to immigration status. Both the 1908 Old Age Pensions Act and the 1911 National Insurance Act contained residency and nationality requirement. By 1925 there was already a whole series of welfare statutes that linked entitlement to immigration status (Cohen 1996). Opposition to the nexus between welfare and immigration status has been voiced from a very early stage by those denied welfare. The *Jewish Chronicle* of 25 July 1919 reported the Board of Deputies sending a delegation to the Committee of Inquiry which was investigating the Old Age Pensions Act. This was to criticise the linking of a citizenship criterion to pension entitlement which had existed since the first Old Age Pensions Act. By 1925 the *Chronicle* was reporting Joseph Prag, a member of the Board of Deputies, as saying that 'This country in its treatment of aliens has been making a descent to Avernus, beginning with its restriction of alien immigration and from then proceeding to impose liabilities on aliens already here'. This was said specifically in relation to the London County Council linking both its education scholarships and its council housing to immigration status.

Within recent times the new poor law introduced by the 1999 legislation, and in particular the voucher scheme, has been condemned by many trade unions. The *Guardian* of 28 and 29 September 2000 reported the Transport and General Workers Union (TGWU) condemning the scheme at the Labour Party conference. The TGWU made public a dossier at the conference, used to lobby ministers for an end to the scheme, including its link to racial harassment. This, according to the *Guardian*, followed a resolution at the Trades Union Congress unanimously opposing the scheme.

The sharpest form of opposition to immigration-linked welfare provisions has undoubtedly been the protests mounted by asylum seekers against the new poor law. The examples given at the start of this chapter all involve direct and collective action against the new scheme. However, there is no evidence prior to 1945 of workers within welfare protesting the link between entitlements and status. Such protests have occurred, albeit spasmodically, post-1945. For instance 1982 saw the introduction of the NHS (Charges to Overseas Visitors) Regulations. These, with certain exceptions, made availability of free hospital treatment dependent upon residency status. Various unions opposed this, for instance NALGO and NUPE.[8] In particular, The Confederation of Health Service Employees (COHSE), the health workers union, came out against the regulations and submitted its comments in a document (5/81) to the DHSS. The *Guardian* of 19 October 1981 reported the General Secretary of COHSE as saying that his members 'will not act as immigration officers'. There are also examples of welfare workers organising outside of the trade union structures. For instance, in 1985 benefit workers established the Committee for Non-Racist Benefits.

Non-compliance in status assessment

Within the continuum of opposition there remains the core issue of what resistance, if any, has been conducted by welfare workers within the workplace? The highest form of opposition from within the system would be a refusal to comply with any assessment of immigration status prior to the dispensing of benefits. This would be the workplace equivalent of anti-deportation campaigns – as these campaigns essentially refuse to comply with the state's definition of who can come or remain here. Workplace non-compliance becomes a sensible option only when backed by union organisation. Otherwise individual workers are vulnerable. However unions have been reluctant or ambiguous in supporting a position of non-compliance. UNISON, the local authority workers' union and an amalgamation of NALGO, NUPE and COHSE, is an example. *Focus*, the union's journal, reported the debate on a resolution urging non-compliance at its 1996 annual delegate conference (28 June 1996). One delegate said 'Our members are being asked to act as immigration officers. It's not a job they applied to do!' The resolution was defeated.

UNISON's National Executive Committee (NEC) has consistently and successfully sought to amend any resolution at national delegate conferences which contains a reference to non-compliance or non-cooperation. An example was a resolution against the 1996 Asylum and Immigration Act[9] submitted by the National Black Members Committee to the union's 1998 conference. The 1996 Act contained various provisions linking entitlement to status. An NEC amendment deleting all reference to non-cooperation was carried. The Black Members' resolution was itself somewhat strange and contradictory. It states 'many black members have successfully ignored the implementation of the Act and . . . many authorities, health bodies and others are *de facto* rendering the Act unworkable'. Unfortunately there is very little evidence for this. The resolution then 'commends the action of these workers and notes with concern that if found out they could be disciplined'. It asks quite correctly, that the union 'provide guidance to members and branches on protecting members caught not cooperating with the Act's provisions'. However it also 'believes that to highlight a policy of non-cooperation could jeopardise these black workers' efforts'. It is not a sustainable position to support individual members in refusing to comply with legislation, whilst at the same time to deny that this non-compliance should be union policy and should somehow take place in secret.

More positive union responses

UNISON is itself contradictory on the question of non-cooperation/non-compliance. There are examples at a national level where it has been positive on the question. For instance the same issue of *Focus* which reported the defeat at the 1996 conference on non-cooperation, also reported the conference supporting 'a major publicity campaign in support of non-cooperation'. A subsequent issue of *Focus*, though falling short of recommending non-compliance, did try to put some restraint on status investigation (19 July 1996). It advised that 'branches should demand a full risk assessment where staff are asked to carry out checks on the immigration status of service users'. The same issue of *Focus* also discussed what position its members should take towards the implementation of employer sanctions. Employer sanctions were introduced by the 1996 Asylum and Immigration Act. They penalise employers for hiring workers ineligible for employment because of their immigration status. They effectively transform bosses into agents of immigration control. Just as seriously, they also implicate fellow-workers, for instance in personnel departments, who are asked to investigate status. *Focus* stated: 'Branches have been issued with advice on how to resist any attempts to force members to carry out immigration checks . . . branches should ask employers to refuse to implement checks on the immigration status of employees' (19 July 1996).

Suggested future strategies for non-compliance

Certain unions, because of their particular industrial or commercial ██████are in a key strategic position to implement a policy of non-compliance. USDAW, the shop-workers' union, is an example. Shop-workers could refuse to accept vouchers under the scheme introduced in the 1999 legislation – pressurising the government to reintroduce full, monetary-based, benefits for asylum seekers and others subject to controls.

Non-compliance is inevitably a high-risk option for workers, even where supported by their union. The most effective way to eliminate the risk is to gain the support of management in non-compliance. This itself will be possible, if at all, only through union organisation and anti-racist agitation. It is difficult to envisage management within certain agencies ever adopting such a stance – particularly management within government-controlled bodies such as the Benefits Agency. However other organisations may be open to the adoption of a policy of non-compliance. One example is National Health Trusts. As has been seen, hospitals are legally obliged to levy charges for hospital treatment based on residency status. However, research has shown that many hospitals simply do not comply, even though this non-compliance is not a consequence of objection in principle, but of objection against the bureaucracy involved (Cohen *et al.* 1997).

It may also be possible to break councils from the investigation of immigration status. Following the 1999 Immigration and Asylum Act a new, if minor, industry has been created within local authorities. This has been established to help administer the poor law housing dispersal scheme for asylum seekers. This has made even more council workers complicit in a system of immigration-linked welfare. Many councillors and perhaps many council workers regard this new scheme as being in some way benevolent in that it is providing accommodation for asylum seekers. However it is a malevolent scheme. It is based on forced dispersal within a cashless economy where asylum seekers are given vouchers at 70 per cent income support level. The only principled position is for local councils to refuse to cooperate with this poor law and by this non-cooperation politically force the government to restore all benefits and housing rights to asylum seekers and others subject to controls. Local authorities do not exist outside of the state. They are part of it. However, it is sometimes possible to engender splits between the local and national state. There have been historic examples of this in respect to immigration controls. For instance, during the period 1979–1997 there was increasing tightening of controls by the Tory Government whilst at the same time at least some Labour-controlled local authorities, such as Manchester, were supporting and helping finance anti-deportation campaigns (Cohen 2001). Workers, their unions and organisations opposed to immigration controls should campaign for local authorities to refuse cooperation with the dispersal scheme.

No information to be given to Home Office

There is a flip-side to the investigation of immigration status for the purposes of welfare entitlement. This is the pressure on workers or on designated workers to report any allegedly unlawful status to the Home Office – with the pressure coming from the Home Office itself. For instance, in October 1996 the Immigration and Nationality Directorate issued its guidelines *Home Office Circular to Local Authorities in Great Britain. Exchange of information with the Immigration and Nationality Directorate (IND) of the Home Office.* The circular's purpose was: 'to invite local authorities to use facilities offered by the IND in identifying claimants who may be ineligible for a benefit or service by virtue of their immigration status; and to encourage local authorities to pass information to the IND about suspected immigration offenders'. It ought to be fundamental trade union policy that its members never act as Home Office informers. Indeed unions should exercise disciplinary powers, including the power of exclusion, over members who act as informers. However, the leadership of unions has been reluctant to sanction even this form of non-cooperation. For example, the Manchester Community Health Branch submitted a resolution to the 1998 UNISON health workers' conference. This condemned the linking of hospital treatment to immigration status and resolved that if health workers were asked to give information on status to the Home Office 'they should be urged to refuse to cooperate and should be supported by UNISON if they suffer any repercussions as a consequence'. UNISON's Health Care Service Group Executive successfully amended the resolution by deleting this reference to non-cooperation on informing.

How the ideology can influence the action

A further issue referred to previously needs to be discussed. This is whether, and if so in what way, the divergent ideological positions of advocacy of no controls compared to advocacy of 'fair' controls may lead to divergent courses of political action. Two initial points can be made. First it is important to make a distinction within the camp of those arguing for the possibility and desirability of 'fair' controls. When this position is proposed by a Labour Government enacting laws such as the 1999 Immigration and Asylum Act, then it is difficult to believe its authenticity other than as a transparent shield behind which the law is being tightened. This lack of authenticity is self-evident, both in the title and the content of the government white paper, 'Fairer, Faster and Firmer', (Home Office 1998) issued prior to the 1999 legislation. On the other hand there are many people, including many Labour Party members, who genuinely consider there can and should be 'fair' controls. Second, it is quite possible for those of different political ideologies to embark on joint political action. Human progress would be limited if this were not the case. However there are important political consequences that flow logically from a position of *no* controls, which do not flow, or necessarily flow from a genuinely held position of 'fair' controls. Below are particular examples.

First, all immigration cases are politically of equal 'merit'. Anyone wishing to come or remain here should be supported, irrespective of the facts of the case. A critical example of this is the need to support prisoners under threat of deportation following a criminal conviction. A demand for 'fair' controls assumes only 'fair' cases should be supported.

Second, in whatever way cases are presented to the Home Office, campaigns against deportation should base themselves publicly, not on pity or on 'compassion', but on solidarity with those threatened with expulsion. Emphasising the 'compassionate' circumstances of a case simply reinforces the assumption that the right to stay here depends on proof of 'exceptional' circumstances.

Third, any demand for 'fair' controls leaves untouched and even unmentioned the whole issue of immigration-linked welfare. The demand for no controls means rolling back the entire welfare system to its inception and reformulating it, devoid of all reference to immigration, citizenship or residency status. It means fighting to break the link between welfare and nationalism.

Fourth, antagonism to all controls, owing to their inherent racism, means that compliance is offensive to all anti-racist practice.

Linking resistance from without and resistance from within

The original *In and Against The State* publication advocated an alliance of users/consumers of welfare and workers within welfare. This unity is also the way forward within the context of immigration-defined welfare. There have been occasional attempts to cement such an alliance, but this has never really progressed beyond propaganda. These attempts have often been initiated by anti-deportation campaigns where the withholding of benefits from those under threat of expulsion has been correctly interpreted as an effort to starve them out of the country. Several such cases and campaigns occurred in the early 1980s. For instance, Parveen Khan, who came to the UK to join her husband, was deprived of both supplementary benefit (income support) and child benefit because of the immigration status of her husband who was accused of being an unlawful entrant. This deprivation was eventually held to be wrong in law (though today with the tightening of the rules the courts may come to a different conclusion). Parveen and her husband also won their campaign to stay here. This is recorded in a Runnymede Trust pamphlet, *Deportations and Removals* (Gordon 1984). One of the activities of the campaign was to call for a national day of action consisting of pickets outside (then) DHSS offices protesting the link between immigration status and benefit entitlement. This occurred in various cities. However, attempts to elicit the support of DHSS workers through their unions to encourage them to join the pickets, met with little positive response.

Nonetheless the need for a political alliance between those threatened by immigration controls and workers within welfare is now more vital than ever before. This is because of the near-universal identification of welfare entitlements and immigration status. It is imperative that this alliance involves those unions that organise welfare workers, otherwise the latter will be left exposed and powerless. Such an alliance represents the convergence of resistance, both in and against the state, to the convergence of welfare controls and immigration controls.

Notes

1 The community care and children legislation became linked to immigration status by the 1999 Immigration and Asylum Act.
2 In fact the NALGO resolution contained a central if common ambiguity. It called for 'the elimination of racist immigration controls'. This suggests either all controls are racist or that racism can be eliminated from controls whilst still leaving controls intact.
3 There was no 1981 Immigration Act. Todd meant the 1981 British Nationality Act.

4 The Act became operative on 1 January 1906, and its appeal provisions were
   repealed by the 1914 Aliens Amendment Act.
5 London's book is the latest and most authoritative documentation of how
   Britain closed its borders to Jewish refugee victims of Nazism. It details the
   private communications and deputations to ministers by Jewish refugee
   organisations. However, there seems to have been no public protest. At the
   same time (and with the exception of the Quakers) activity for the entry of
   Jewish refugees by non-Jewish organisations, in particular the trade unions,
   whether private or public, seem to have been virtually non-existent.
   According to London, 'political refugees held a special attention for the
   Left, the Labour Party and trade union circles. These groups responded
   sympathetically to the plight of the left-wing opposition in Germany and
   Austria, and felt concern over the fate of social democratic opponents of
   German claims to Czechoslovakia's territory. The British Left had been
   actively involved in the Spanish Civil War and aid to Spanish refugees.
   Eleanor Rathbone MP was tirelessly active on behalf of refugees from both
   political and racial persecution. Generally however, the Left tended to focus
   on political cases'.
6 Claudia Jones, a communist, had herself been deported from the USA
   because of her political beliefs and activities.
7 But note also the campaign against deportation of an Italian, Franco
   Caprino, who was threatened with deportation because of trade union
   activities.
8 *Guardian* 15 April 1981 and 13 October 1981. For full details of this opposition see Cohen (1982).
9 Wrongly called the Immigration and Asylum Act.

References

Cohen, S. (1982) *From Ill Treatment to No Treatment*, Manchester: Manchester
   Law Centre.
—— (1995) *Workers' Control, Not Immigration Controls*, Manchester: Greater
   Manchester Immigration Aid Unit.
—— (1996) *Still Struggling After All These Years*, Manchester: Greater
   Manchester Immigration Aid Unit.
—— (1996) 'Anti-semitism, immigration controls and the welfare state', in D.
   Taylor (ed.) *Critical Social Policy: a reader*, London: Sage, pp 27–47.
—— (2000) 'Never mind the racism – feel the quality', *Immigration and
   Nationality Law and Practice*, 14(4): 223–226.
—— (2001) *Immigration Controls, the Family and the Welfare State*, London:
   Jessica Kingsley Publishers.
Cohen, S., Hayes, D., Humphries, B. and Sime, C. (1997) *Immigration and
   Health: a survey of NHS Trusts and GP Practices*, Manchester: Greater
   Manchester Immigration Aid Unit and Manchester Metropolitan
   University.
Gordon, P. (1984) *Deportations and Removals*, London: Runnymede Trust.
Hayter, T. (2000) *Open Borders: the case against immigration controls*, London:
   Pluto Press.

Home Office (1998) *Fairer, Faster and Firmer: a modern approach to immigration and asylum*, Cm. 4018, London: HMSO.

London, L. (1999) *Whitehall and the Jews, 1933–1948: British immigration policy and the Holocaust*, Cambridge: Cambridge University Press.

London to Edinburgh Weekend Return Group (1979) *In and Against the State*, London: Pluto Press.

Spencer, S. (1994) *Subjects and Citizens*, London: Institute for Public Policy Research.

Index

voucher scheme for asylum seekers
26, 43, 111–17, 122, 131, 146, 154,
176, 178, 191, 202, 226, 229
voucher system for entry to the UK
48

Wandsworth, London Borough of
132
Webb, Sidney and Beatrice   37
Webber, F.   19, 95, 110
welcoming of immigrants   217–18
welfare reforms   37–8, 60
welfare state, the   x, 2, 22–4, 215
welfare workers, resistance by
227–32
West Indian Gazette   225
West Indian Workers' Association
225
Westminster, London Borough of
136
Williams of Mostyn, Lord   192

Williams, Herbert   33
Wilson, Cathcart   32
Windrush   50
work permits   47, 54, 56
working class migrants   48–9, 52
Working Families Tax Credit   5
World Bank   54–5
World Trade Organisation   25
Wythenshawe Hospital   56

xenophobia   14

Yellowlees Report (1980)   39
Young, Jock   42
Younge, Gary   20
Yuval-Davis, N.   214–15

Zetter, R.   110
Zimmerman, K.F.   205
Zwickau   220